AF785725

Franz Frühwald/D. Eric Blackwell (eds.)

Atlas of Color-Coded Doppler Sonography

Vascular and Soft Tissue Structures of the Upper Extremity, Thoracic Outlet and Neck

Springer-Verlag Wien GmbH

Dr. Franz X. J. Frühwald
Department of Radiology, University of Vienna Medical School, and Institute of Diagnostic Imaging, St. Pölten, Austria

Dr. D. Eric Blackwell
Division of Ultrasound, Department of Radiology, Texas Tech University Medical School, Texas, U.S.A.

This work is subject to copyright.
All rights are reserved, whether the whole or part of the material is concerned, specifically those of translation, reprinting, re-use of illustrations, broadcasting, reproduction by photocopying machines or similar means, and storage in data banks.
© 1992 by Springer-Verlag Wien
Originally published by Springer-Verlag/Wien in 1992

Softcover reprint of the hardcover 1st edition 1992
Printed on acid-free paper

With 204 partly coloured Figures and 4 Drawings

Cover-design: T. Erben, Wien

Product Liability: The publisher can give no guarantee for information about drug dosage and application thereof contained in this book. In every individual case the respective user must check its accuracy by consulting other pharmaceutical literature. The use of registered names, trademarks, etc. in this publication does not imply, even in the absence of a specific statement, that such names are exempt from the relevant protective laws and regulations and therefore free for general use.

Library of Congress Cataloging-in-Publication Data. Atlas of color coded doppler sonography : vascular and soft tissue structures of the upper extremity, thoracic outlet and neck / Franz X. J. Frühwald, D. Eric Blackwell (eds.). p. cm. ISBN-13:978-3-7091-9197-2
1. Extremities, Upper–Blood-vessels–Ultrasonic imaging–Atlases. 2. Neck–Blood-vessels–Ultrasonic imaging–Atlases. 3. Doppler ultrasonography–Atlases. I. Frühwald, Franz X. J., 1957– . [DNLM: 1. Arm–blood supply–atlases. 2. Arm–ultrasonography–atlases. 3. Neck–blood supply–atlases. 4. Neck–ultrasonography–atlases. 5. Thoracic Arteries–atlases. 6. Thoracic Arteries–ultrasonography–atlases. 7. Thoracic Nerves–blood supply–atlases. 8. Thoracic Nerves–ultrasonography–atlases. 9. Ultrasonography–methods–atlases. WE 17 A8795]
QM548.A75 1992. 611′.97–dc20. DNLM/DLC. 92-2332

ISBN 978-3-7091-9197-2 ISBN 978-3-7091-9195-8 (eBook)
DOI 10.1007/978-3-7091-9195-8

Foreword

For those of us who have been associated with the field of ultrasound imaging of the arterial system since its infancy, this contribution by Frühwald and Blackwell provides the source where the results of over 30 years of hard-won advances can be found. The editors and contributors summarize this burgeoning field in their lucidly written, interesting, and accurate treatise. Beginning with chapters on physical principles and technical considerations, including how to adjust equipment for best images, they consider forthwith carotid and vertebral disease in two outstanding chapters with color images of startling definition. Also included are diagrams in which vascular structures are clearly related to well-labeled anatomical landmarks. No other atlas contains the quality of color images and graphic displays which these two editors have compiled.

Now that surgical remediation of stenosis of the extracranial carotid and, perhaps, also the vertebral arteries has been demonstrated effective there will undoubtedly be an explosion in the use of this advanced technology to identify appropriate patients and to follow lesions longitudinally over time. To accomplish this, high-quality images made by skilled sonographers are the vital component and this book sets standards in this domain.

To this material, they have added chapters on extremity and thyroid imaging and closing chapters on diseases of veins and dialysis fistulas. Perhaps only specialists will be interested in these topics but, nevertheless, in a compendium dealing with vascular imaging, all of the areas must be included and these chapters will provide useful information. In their depictions of the physiologic changes which can occur, their line drawings are a welcome addition to the images taken from the video screen.

It is particularly gratifying to those of us who have been involved in the field since its inception to see the giant strides that technologic development and image quality have made on both sides of the Atlantic. This collaboration brings the best of European and American knowledge together in a clearly written, understandable text. Of special note is the quality of the chapter on the vertebral artery system which will ensure that this atlas has a special place as a reference for technicians and physicians interested in the cerebral circulation.

It is my special pride that one of the editors (D. E. Blackwell) is a graduate of my training program where he performed in an outstanding manner, subsequent to which he acquired the skills which he has put to such good use in bringing to readers of the English version of this book a clear rendering of the extensive work of his colleagues in Vienna, interwoven with the latest information from research centers in the United States.

James F. Toole, M.D. March, 1992
Teagle Professor and Chairman Emeritus,
Department of Neurology
Director, Stroke Research Center
The Bowman Gray School of Medicine of
Wake Forest University
Winston-Salem, North Carolina

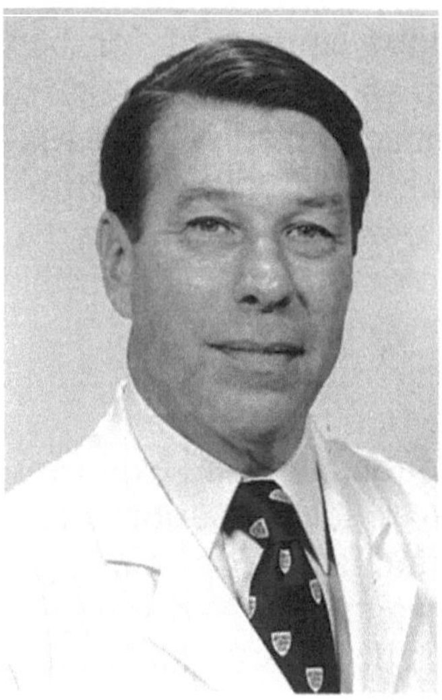

Prof. James F. Tool is Member of numerous scientific societies, committees and associations. Besides other functions he served as President of the American Neurological Association (1983–1985), from 1982 to 1992 in different functions in the Board of the World Federation of Neurology and is since 1992 President of the American Society of Neuroimaging. He also is editor of numerous textbooks and of the Journal of Neurological Sciences as well as of World Neurology and he serves in the editorial boards of numerous scientific Journals.
He has published more than 200 scientific papers.

Preface

When the editors and authors first considered the possibility of putting together this atlas of color Doppler ultrasound, several specific goals were formulated. The first was to produce a book with the highest possible quality of color reproduction, working almost entirely from transparencies created directly from the ultrasound scanning unit using a slide recorder. We are grateful to Springer-Verlag for the continued attention to detail which has resulted in extremely high-quality and accurate color rendition in the published plates, an effort which was pursued with no imposed limit on the costs involved.

A second goal was to provide line drawings and other graphic illustrations to lend clarity to the explanations of anatomic relationships and scan techniques. Credit for all of these diagrams goes to one of the authors, Dr. Peter Hübsch.

Our third goal was to bring together in one reference work not only the most recent findings from clinical studies done on state-of-the-art equipment but also an overview of related articles from the world literature and some historical context for each type of procedure. Extensive bibliographic listings have been created for each chapter.

Much of the credit for organizing the entire project must be given to Dr. Franz Frühwald who not only contributed material to several of the chapters but also coordinated the efforts of contributors on both sides of the Atlantic and served as liaison with the publisher.

This atlas represents a new approach to international publishing, with one set of very expensive color plates in the English edition supplemented by complete French and German translations of the text included in the same volume. This reflects both the increasing unity of economic effort in the European community and the realities of trying to minimize cost-per-book by addressing a larger total market with books for even relatively small medical subspecialty areas. Credit is given to Dr. D. Eric Blackwell (Texas Tech University School of Medicine) for editing the English edition, to Dr. Michel Dauzat (Université de Nimes, France) and Dr. Michel Lafortune (Université de Montreal, Canada) for the excellent French translation, and to Dr. Frühwald for the final version in German.

Most of the color images in the atlas are from studies performed with color Doppler scanners manufactured by Acuson. The remaining color scans are from instruments by Advanced Technology Laboratories, Toshiba, and Philips.

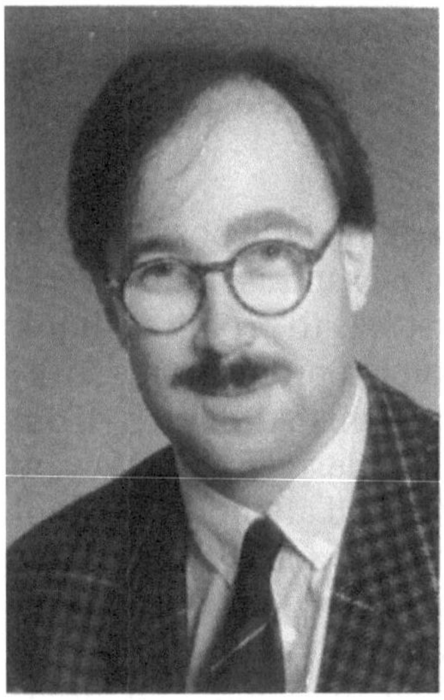

Franz X. J. Frühwald, M.D.

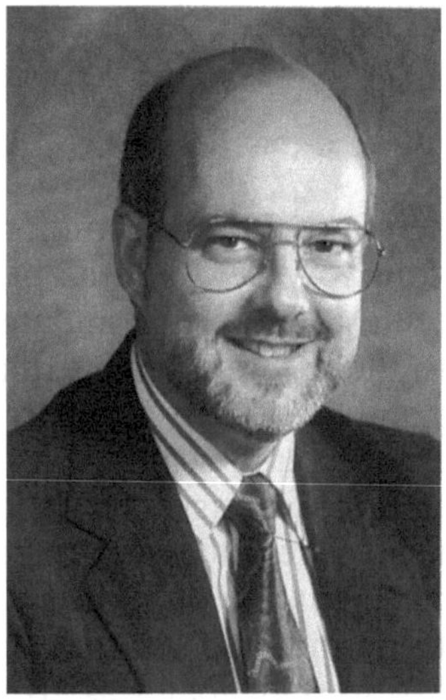

D. Eric Blackwell, M.D.

Contents

Contributors

Franz X. J. Frühwald, M.D., Assistant Professor of Radiology, University of Vienna and Chief of the Institute of Diagnostic Imaging, St. Pölten, Austria

D. Eric Blackwell, M.D., Professor of Radiology and Chief, Division of Ultrasound, Texas Tech University School of Medicine, Lubbock, Texas, U.S.A.

Siegfried Trattnig, M.D., Lecturer, Department of Radiology, University of Vienna, Austria

Peter Hübsch, M.D., Lecturer, Department of Radiology, University of Vienna, Austria

1
CCDS: Physical principles and technical considerations

F. Frühwald and D. E. Blackwell

Introduction

CCDS (color-coded Doppler sonography – also referred to as color Doppler ultrasound or CDU) is a combined ultrasound modality offering blood flow information superimposed on a gray scale picture. Areas within the image which contain flowing blood (or other moving or vibrating tissue or particles – a potential source of artifact) are assigned color-overlay information based on a number of parameters including direction of flow, mean flow velocity, and velocity variance (which can be an indicator of turbulence). Flow toward the transducer is generally encoded as red, flow away from the probe as blue. As velocity increases the assigned color becomes lighter in shade; this often referred to as "color fading" or "decreased color saturation" (Figs. 2, 3). Many CCDS instruments allow introduction of additional color (often green or orange) in areas where marked variation in velocity is encountered (Fig. 9); this can help visually "flag" regions of turbulent flow as are often encountered just distal to an area of stenosis.

Two-dimensional information is gained by high quality realtime gray scale technology. Specially designed multigated pulsed Doppler circuitry (see below) acquires the information used for determination of areas to be color-encoded and can also be used for acquisition of conventional spectral waveforms for analysis and measurement purposes, including determination of *peak* velocity values as well as the *mean* velocity information most commonly used for the color mapping process.

The acquisition of optimal information using a CCDS scanner is not a trivial process due to the large number of variables which must be optimized. A separate chapter titled "CCDS: Optimizing Scan Techniques . . ." is devoted to maximizing the effectiveness and accuracy of CCDS in clinical practice. It gives in-depth consideration to such issues as choosing the optimum scan angle for gray scale imaging and for color and duplex Doppler, proper choice of power and sensitivity settings, quality control, and methods of image capture for documentation and long-term storage. All of these issues must be well understood if operator-dependent errors in diagnosis are to be avoided.

The sections which follow will provide a physical and historical context for the understanding of CCDS. A brief review of the basic physics underlying the Doppler principle will be followed by discussions of continuous wave (CW) Doppler, pulsed Doppler and duplex scanners and the design and technical differences between pulsed and CW systems, and finally an overview of system design considerations for CCDS scanners. For in-depth information on these topics the reader is encouraged to consult the excellent references cited at the end of the chapter.

The Doppler principle

Credit for the first written account of the physical principle that waves moving between an observer and a source will be stretched (reduced in frequency) or compressed (increased in frequency) if there is relative motion between the source and observer is given to Christian Andreas Doppler (Eden, 1990). His work was oriented toward astrophysics and the understanding of red-shifted light waves from celestial objects moving away from observers on earth. The concept is readily applicable to wave behavior for sound at or above the range of human hearing as well. If source and observer are *not* moving relative to each other a sequence of waves will be heard by the observer at the same pitch generated at the source. If the two are moving closer together the observer will encounter each passing wave at a faster rate and will perceive an increase in pitch relative to the source; if relative motion of the two is away from each other then fewer waves per unit time will be encountered and a lower pitch will be noted by the observer. If the observed frequency value is subtracted from the actual (source) frequency the resulting value, known as the Doppler shift frequency, can be used to determine how fast the observer and source are moving toward or away from each other. Mathematically this can be expressed in somewhat simplified form by the following equation:

$$f_D = 2\,f_0\,v\cos\theta/c$$

where f_D is the Doppler frequency shift, f_0 is the incident frequency, v is the flow velocity, c is the speed of sound in human tissue, and theta is the angle between the path of the central ultrasound beam and the direction of flow (Burns, 1987; Atkinson, 1982; Taylor, 1990). The factor of 2 on the right side of the equation reflects the fact that both send time and receive time must be taken into consideration. As will be discussed in the following section, f_D happens to fall into the frequency range of human hearing for incident (transmit) frequency values in the 3–10 MHz range and velocity values such as those associated with moving structures in the heart or erythrocytes propelled in the moving blood stream; this was of practical importance in the earliest applications of continuous wave Doppler instruments to analysis of human physiology.

Continuous wave (CW) Doppler instruments

The earliest Doppler instruments applied to medical use were of the type known as continuous wave (CW) Doppler flow detectors or “Doppler stethoscopes”. Typically these units had two transducer elements: one would generate ultrasound waves continuously and the second served to receive returning waves and convert these to small electrical pulses which could then be amplified and further processed. The transmitting or "send" frequency was usually in the 3 to 10 MHz range. It was found that for physiologic motion in the body (moving elements in the blood or moving tissues in the heart) the Doppler shift frequency values (transmit frequency minus returning shifted frequency) were in the range of human hearing (Taylor, 1990; Merritt, 1991). These could be amplified and sent to a speaker or set of headphones; "processing" of the information consisted of interpretation of the sounds by a skilled sonographer or physician. Even with the most advanced generation of Doppler instruments this direct auditory input remains an important guiding factor in many examinations. The addition of quadrature detection circuitry to these early CW units added the important ability to determine *direction* of flow; hard-copy devices such as strip chart recorders were also added making it possible to document frequency (or velocity) changes vs. time. Much attention was then devoted to interpretation of the magnitude and shape changes of the resulting patterns as related to underlying vascular properties such as high- or low-resistance to flow, focal or generalized vessel narrowing, or cardiac valvular abnormalities.

CW Doppler instruments had the advantage of being simple in design and inexpensive to manufacture. They were usually small units which could be easily moved to the patient bedside; later units were battery powered and could literally be carried in a pocket. Applications quickly developed in obstetrics (for rapid determination of viability in early pregnancy and for evaluation of fetal heart rate and umbilical artery flow patterns later in pregnancy) and in vascular surgery, where skilled observers could gain a large amount of helpful information regarding arterial stenosis or venous flow properties previously requiring angiography. Several disadvantages quickly became apparent, however. Perhaps the most significant of these was that CW units return Doppler-shift information from the entire area insonated. If several vascular structures at different depths were encountered then the returning Doppler information was a composite of all the motion occurring in all the vessels. This problem could be somewhat overcome with directional CW Doppler instruments since the most common vascular pattern encountered in the neck or extremities is an artery paired with a vein; the proper choice of scan angle could give a recorded pattern with venous signals "below the baseline" and arterial signals above it. Even in this situation, analysis of arterial patterns such as flow reversal in diastole was often difficult or impossible. Another problem arose from the lack of precise knowledge of the angle of insonation (the angle between the wavefront generated by the Doppler unit and the direction of flow in the vessel being evaluated). This angle is important in accurate calculation of Doppler shift frequency and flow velocity values, which vary with the cosine of the angle of insonation: a maximum cosine value of 1 at 0 degrees (directly in line with the moving targets) and a cosine value of 0 at 90 degrees to the path of motion. The need for a B-scan image to demonstrate the direction of underlying vessels being evaluated by Doppler techniques and to demonstrate plaque and/or thrombus within the vessels was an important driving force in the development of duplex (i.e. both imaging and Doppler) ultrasound instruments, which will be discussed in the following section.

Pulsed Doppler and duplex scanners

The next evolutionary step in medical application of Doppler ultrasound came with the introduction of pulsed Doppler instruments. These generally used the same transducer for sending and receiving of ultrasound in discrete pulse "packets" rather than in a continuous stream. A major advantage gained by this approach is the ability to define a single small area of interest along the path of the beam for sampling instead of detecting all moving structures in the insonated area (Fig. 1 a). By varying the elapsed time between sending and "listening" a small sample volume of some desired axial length can be effectively established within the gray-scale 2-D image at some desired distance from the skin surface (as noted below, the non-axial dimension of the sample volume is established by *focal properties* of the transducer). In anatomic settings where several vascular structures lie in close proximity, such an instrument can selectively sample flow properties from each rather than presenting a composite flow pattern from all the vessels. The same selectivity can be applied to evaluation of flow at discrete points along the course of a single vessel as well, allowing sampling of flow at a point of maximal stenosis as well as proximal and distal to the stenotic area. The exact size of the sampled area depends upon the number of "pulse packets" transmitted in each sequence (this establishes the distance in the axis of the beam which will be sampled) and upon focal characteristics of the beam; the more narrowly focused the beam the smaller the dimension of the sampled volume at right angles to the beam path (Mitchell, 1990). Focal properties can be manipulated by the use of acoustic lens material at the transducer surface and/or choice of transmit and receive patterns in multi-element phased array transducers. Generally the operator of the unit will have more control over axial sample volume size than over the size of the non-axial dimension. Multiple range gates can be assigned to a single scan line (Fig. 1 b) by sampling the returning ultrasound impulses at several intervals; this technique is sometimes used to allow simultaneous display of several structures of interest in M-mode (usually cardiac) scans.

As might be expected, pulsed Doppler systems also have disadvantages. The most important one is related to the fact that flow properties in the targeted vessel must be calculated from a series of individual samples with a small but potentially significant "gap" in time between each. If the actual rate of change in the movement of the "targets" is high compared to the interval between samples a problem known as "aliasing" can occur. This problem does not occur with CW Doppler units since they employ a continuous stream of samples without time gaps. For this reason some pulsed Doppler scanning instruments also have CW Doppler capability for use when high flow velocities are encountered. Aliasing is discussed at some length in the chapter on Optimizing Instrument Settings and in the Carotid Artery chapter; the appearance of aliasing in CCDS images will be considered below.

Color-coded Doppler sonography

If the concept of multiple Doppler gates along a line is extended to include sweeping the multi-gate line through a thin volume of tissue (Fig. 1 c) we have established the underlying concept behind CCDS. Many Doppler data points are then estab-

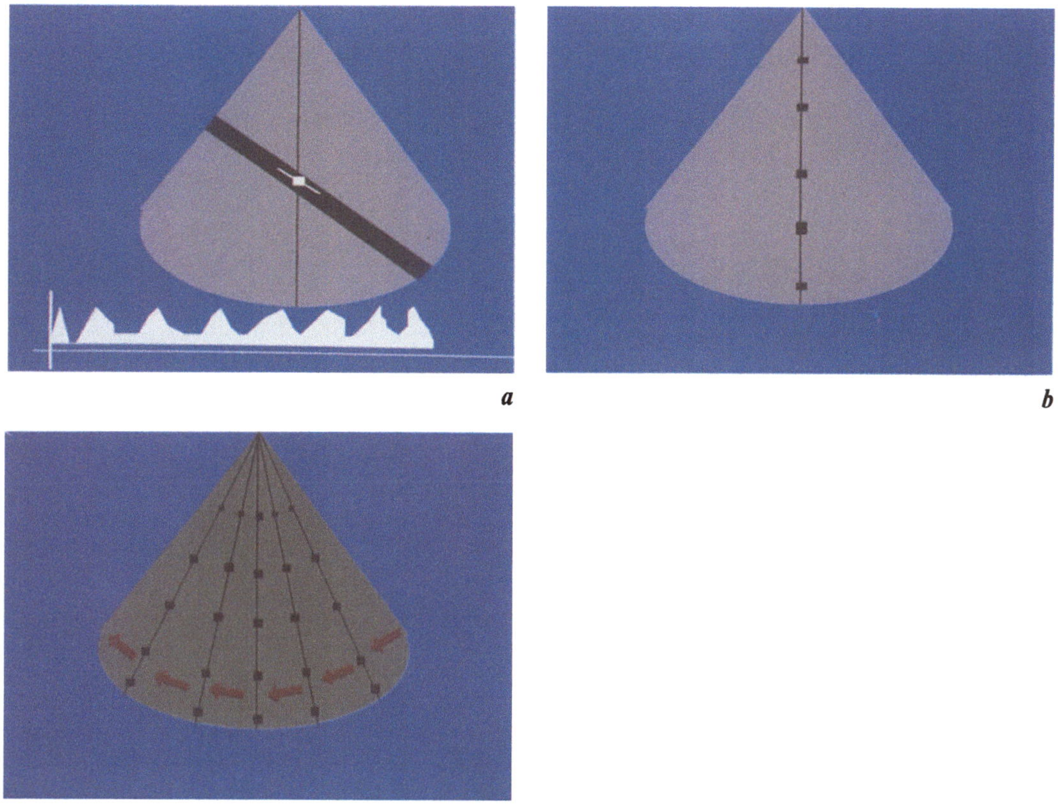

Fig. 1. Diagrams of methods of Doppler data acquisition; ***a*** Spectral Doppler: one range gate is specified (small white rectangle) within a gray scale image; Doppler information from within this small sample volume is displayed as frequency (or velocity) vs. time along the bottom of the image. The white line aligned with the vessel axis allows calculation of the Doppler angle; ***b*** Several range gates along one line allow performance of multigated Doppler (used in M-mode data acquisition and display); ***c*** Several range gates per line can be moved across the gray-scale image to provide Doppler data for a large number of sample points. Several pulses are transmitted for each line of Doppler data; the timing of these pulses establishes the *pulse repetition frequency* (PRF) and the duration of sampling for each line is referred to as the *dwell time*

lished across the entire B-scan image and a "global overview" of blood flow can be obtained. If the Doppler shift information from each sampled point is assigned a *color* based on direction of movement relative to the sound beam, and if the color *intensity* is varied with the mean velocity of flow, then this color-encoded data can be superimposed on the gray scale B-scan image (Fig. 2). The result is a scan which provides a fast method of surveying a large anatomic area for vascular "mapping".

The fact that CCDS is one of the most recent additions to the diagnostic ultrasound "toolbox" relates largely to the extreme complexity of rapid acquisition and manipulation of data from so many individual sample areas. Only the recent exponential increases in computational power at acceptable cost levels, coupled with extensive research and development efforts growing out of the design of duplex Doppler scanners and advanced transducer concepts, have made it possible to bring to market the current generation of color Doppler instruments.

Obtaining data for concurrent gray scale and color Doppler display requires a number of compromises. Optimal scan angle is often 90 degrees to the target

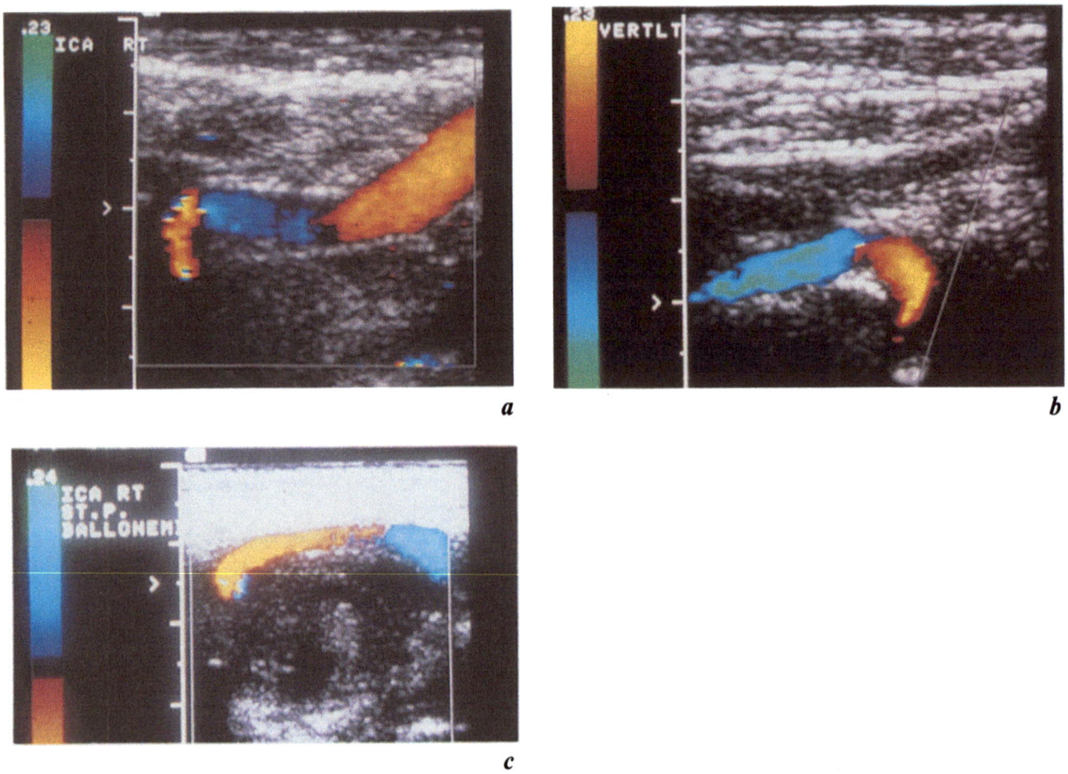

Fig. 2. Color encoding depends on the angle of flow relative to the transducer. In this tortuous carotid artery; ***a*** And normal atlas loop of a vertebral artery; ***b*** Red indicates flow toward the transducer and blue indicates flow away from the transducer. Where the ultrasound beam is perpendicular to the direction of flow a small band devoid of color (black) divides the red- and blue-encoded portions of the vessel. Lighter color saturation in these examples is indicative of areas where the Doppler angle is small as the vessel curves more into the beam path. The curved course of the CCA in illustration; ***c*** Is due to displacement of the vessel by an enlarged ovoid lymph node

surface for B-scan imaging but 30–60 degrees for accurate Doppler-based calculation of velocity. Angles greater than 60 degrees are associated with rapid changes in value of the cosine, rendering frequency and velocity measurements relatively inaccurate. Angles of less than 30 degrees, while ideal from a theoretical standpoint, are often associated with so much reflection from the vessel wall as to be unusable (Taylor, 1990). Usually a single ultrasound pulse per scan line is adequate for gray scale data acquisition, while 3 to 32 pulses may be used for generating Doppler information. Doppler accuracy and adequacy of detection of slow flow velocity increase as more time per line is devoted to data acquisition (increased *dwell time*), but the longer the dwell time the lower the line density and the poorer the depiction of rapidly changing hemodynamics. Maximum gray scale detail is obtained with small pulse "packets" and narrow beam widths, while longer impulse sequences of greater width provide greater Doppler shift resolution. The design evolution of CCDS instruments has involved increasingly ingenious approaches to resolving these conflicting demands.

The *pulse repetition frequency* (PRF) of a Doppler instrument is the rate at which sound wave "packets" are transmitted. This is an extremely important parameter since accurate depth assignment is possible only as long as echoes returning from the target organ are received before the next packet of energy is transmitted. The maximum Doppler shift frequency which can be detected with accuracy is one-half of the PRF value and is referred to as the Nyquist frequency (Mitchell, 1990; Merritt, 1991). When the Nyquist frequency value is exceeded, the result is *aliasing;* in a CCDS image this takes the form of an abrupt shift from light shades of red to light shades of blue (or vice-versa); examples of CCDS aliasing are shown in Figs. 6 and 8. Figure 6a illustrates one type of color flow map where increasing velocity values are indicated by progressive addition of white to the basic color producing a lighter shade of the same color. Figure 6b illustrates an alternative color map where red changes to yellow (and blue to green) with increasing velocity. In Fig. 6c the use of one color (green) to "flag" velocity values above a certain threshold is shown.

The appearance of aliasing should be carefully differentiated from color display of actual flow reversal (as often encountered physiologically in the carotid bulb area where flow separation occurs with deceleration of flow as the vessel lumen becomes wider); true flow reversal is shown by CCDS as a shift from deep red to deep blue (or vice-versa). Between the red- and blue-coded areas there will be a band of black (indicating zero flow velocity). This is illustrated in Figs. 7a, b and c. Figure 8 illustrates both aliasing and flow separation in adjacent areas within a single vessel.

At least one additional color mapping option is available on most CCDS scan units: a "variance" tag; green is often used (Fig. 9). Variance is present when the *range* of frequency shifts within a target area is high; one physiologic situation in which variance is common is the presence of turbulent flow, often encountered just distal to an area of stenosis (Mitchell, 1990). Assigning a distinctly different color to areas of significant variance can be a useful way to "flag" specific vessel segments for detailed evaluation using spectral analysis. The threshold at which turbulence occurs is established by the Reynolds number *Re* as defined by the formula

$$Re = \mathrm{v\,d/viscosity}$$

where v = the blood velocity, d = the lumen diameter, and viscosity = the kinematic viscosity of blood. Turbulence is encountered in physiologic flow systems when *Re* equals about 2300 (Taylor, 1990). It is important to differentiate between turbulence in areas where a pressure drop is present (as encountered distal to a hemodynamically significant vascular stenosis) and turbulence where no pressure drop occurs (as in the carotid bulb where progression from a normal vessel diameter to the even wider bulb area leads to boundary layer separation). The rarity of turbulence in vessels of very small diameter can be understood when the effect of a small value of d in the above equation is noted.

Since most current CCDS instruments utilize *mean velocity* as the basis for color value assignment at each pixel (picture element) some caution must be used when interpreting scan findings. Marked underestimation of peak velocity can occur if careful spectral analysis at selected points of interest is not carried out. Spectral waveform information is derived from the CCDS data using fast Fourier transformation (FFT) algorithms. The resulting graphic representation of frequency (or velocity) values can be analyzed with respect to variations with time of the Doppler frequencies present in the sample volume, the spectrum envelope (representing the maximum frequencies present at any given time), and the spectral width, which is indicative of the *range* of frequencies present (Merritt, 1991). In the presence of

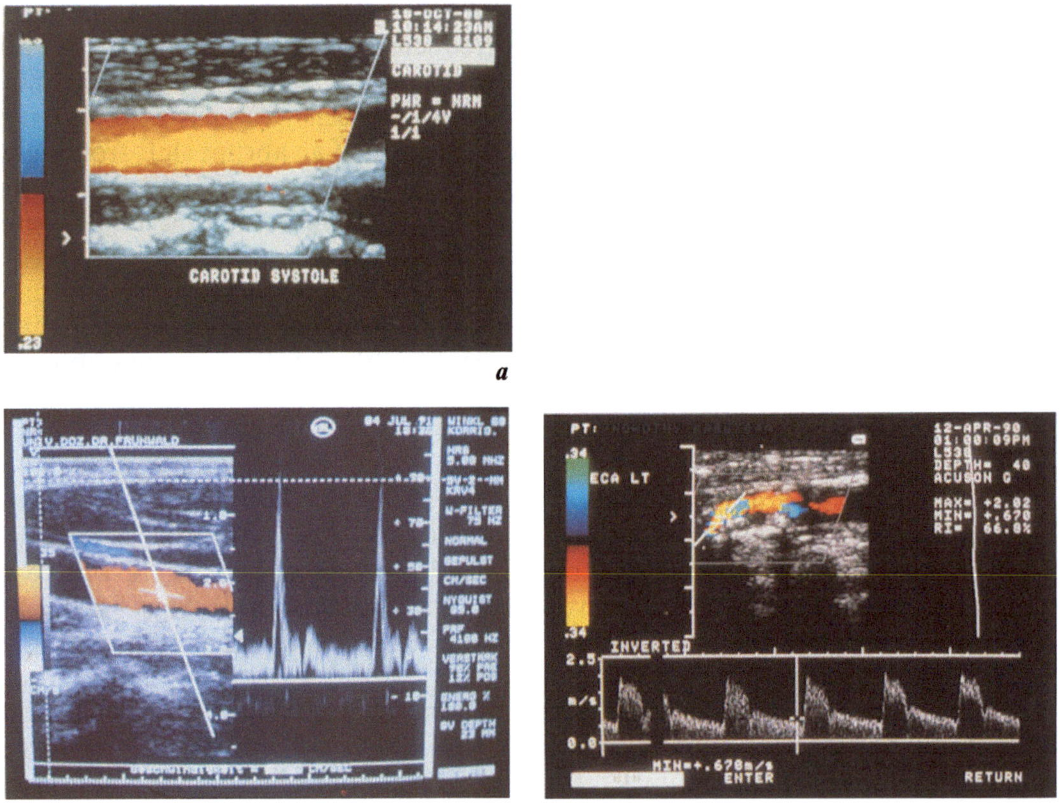

a

b *c*

Fig. 3. Examples of inconstant relationship between frequency (or velocity) values based on the color encoded display (which utilizes values near the mean) and those obtained by spectral waveform analysis (which allows peak values to be obtained); ***a*** Laminar flow in a normal CCA, with lighter color hue centrally consistent with higher flow velocities than at the periphery; ***b*** Normal CCA with laminar flow. Diastolic flow based on color encoding would be about 0.2 m/sec while spectral analysis reveals a peak diastolic velocity in the 0.25 m/sec range; ***c*** In this angiographically confirmed high-grade ICA stenosis, flow velocity of 0.34 m/sec is suggested by color encoding in pale yellow; spectral analysis, however, shows a peak systolic velocity of 2.0 m/sec

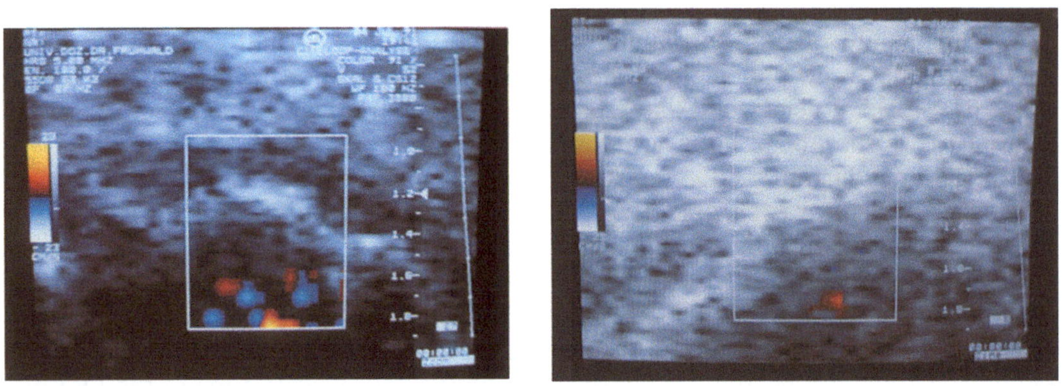

a *b*

Fig. 4. ***a*** Color "noise" in a black area of this image in which gray-shaded areas are free of color display; ***b*** Identical anatomic area shown with increased B-mode gain: color is now suppressed since the area is now dark gray rather than black

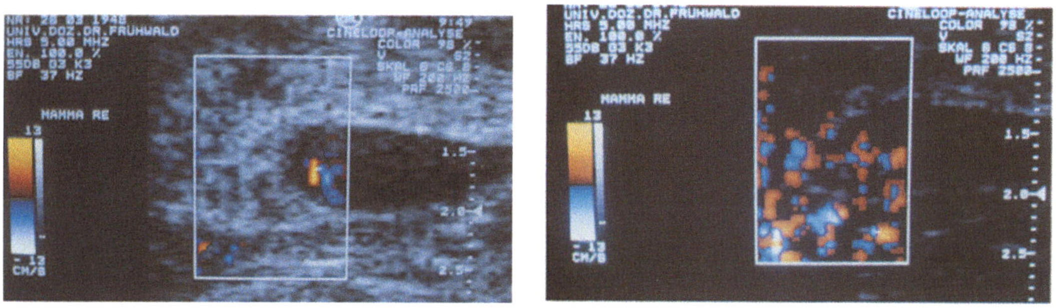

a *b*

Fig. 5. Effect of gray-scale echo intensity on suppression of color noise:
a Color noise artifact shown only in the black area of the image (representing a breast cyst);
b Reduction of B-mode gain without change in color settings allows display of color artifact throughout the image

laminar flow the color-image mean velocity may be fairly close to actual peak velocity values (Fig. 3a, b) while in the presence of wide pulse pressure or turbulence the peak velocity values may greatly exceed the mean values (Fig. 3c). The color-encoded image can provide a rapid method of locating areas of suspected stenosis based on aliasing or variance mapping; the sample volume should then be carefully positioned for acquisition of spectral waveform data at the point of maximum narrowing (and often proximal and distal to the area of stenosis as well). If aliasing is still present when using duplex Doppler then a reduction in PRF, change to a lower Doppler transmit frequency, or an increase in Doppler angle may eliminate the problem and allow display of high-quality waveform patterns for measurement, as discussed in the chapter on Optimizing Instrument Settings. Another approach which can be used on instruments utilizing superheterodyne quadrature demodulation of Doppler signals is to lower the spectral display baseline to provide more "headroom" for display of forward flow (Taylor, 1990); this is at the expense of display room for reversed flow, but in the presence of severe stenosis little or no flow reversal may be present.

Many CCDS scanning units make use of color display strategies which only allow assignment of color to areas of the image with no gray scale information. Color "noise" (a random display of pixels of various colors) may be particularly apparent in images where inadequate gray scale gain is used (Fig. 4a); increasing the gray scale gain will suppress these artifacts (Fig. 4b). A related problem can arise when a non-vascular low-echodensity structure such as the breast cyst shown in Fig. 5a is present: color noise may appear only within the cystic area. The artifactual nature of this pattern can be confirmed by reducing the overall gray scale gain; color noise will then appear in other portions of the image (Fig. 5b). The correct approach to this problem is then to reduce the *color* gain or increase the color reject values while restoring optimal gray scale gain settings.

Numerous processing and image manipulation parameters are used in CCDS imaging units. If separate "sweeps" are used to produce the gray scale and color Doppler image data, any movement of tissue can result in a mis-registration of color data on the B-scan image. This problem can be minimized by interleaving alternate gray scale and color Doppler lines, but the rapid switching required puts heavy demands on the instrument's computer and may lead to a slowing of other

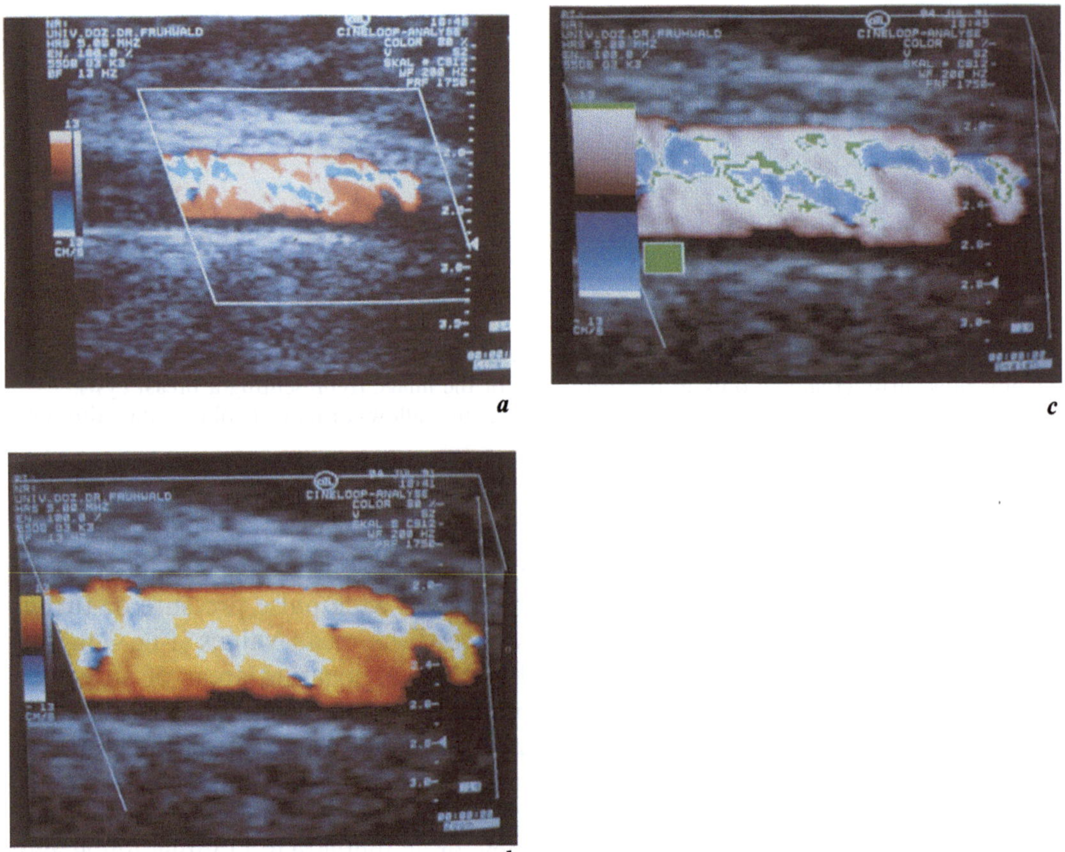

a *c* *b*

Fig. 6. Normal CCA with no abnormality of blood flow; aliasing artifact is due to improper setting of the velocity range to too low a value. Aliasing is easily recognized in ***a*** as a change to opposite color values, from pale red to white to pale blue (without an intervening band of black), occurring when the current velocity range of the system is exceeded by blood flow velocity. The same principle applies when other color maps such as red to yellow and blue to green are used ***b***; green is often used as a third color to "tag" specific flow velocity values ***c***

functions requiring CPU time. The rapid acquisition of Doppler data for color display is usually accomplished using some variation of the technique known as "autocorrelation". This method utilizes successive subtractions of returning wave-forms (each slightly time-shifted relative to the previous one) to remove signal components contributed by non-moving structures; quadrature detection is then applied to the remaining information in order to establish directionality of flow and magnitude of frequency shift (Rubin, 1991).

Several other "smoothing" or "filtering" operations may be employed to provide a more useful and visually pleasing display. Since the CCDS technique is sensitive to any moving structures within the image field, movement of vessel walls or cardiac structures and vibrations of tissue adjacent to areas of pulsatile or turbulent flow can yield very strong Doppler domain signals. All CCDS scanning units employ some method of suppressing the low frequency, high amplitude signals generally arising from pulsatile expansion of vessel walls, giving rise to the commonly used term "wall filter" for this function (Omoto, 1987; Kasai, 1989; Gessert, 1987). Simply setting a cut-off threshold at some low-frequency value is

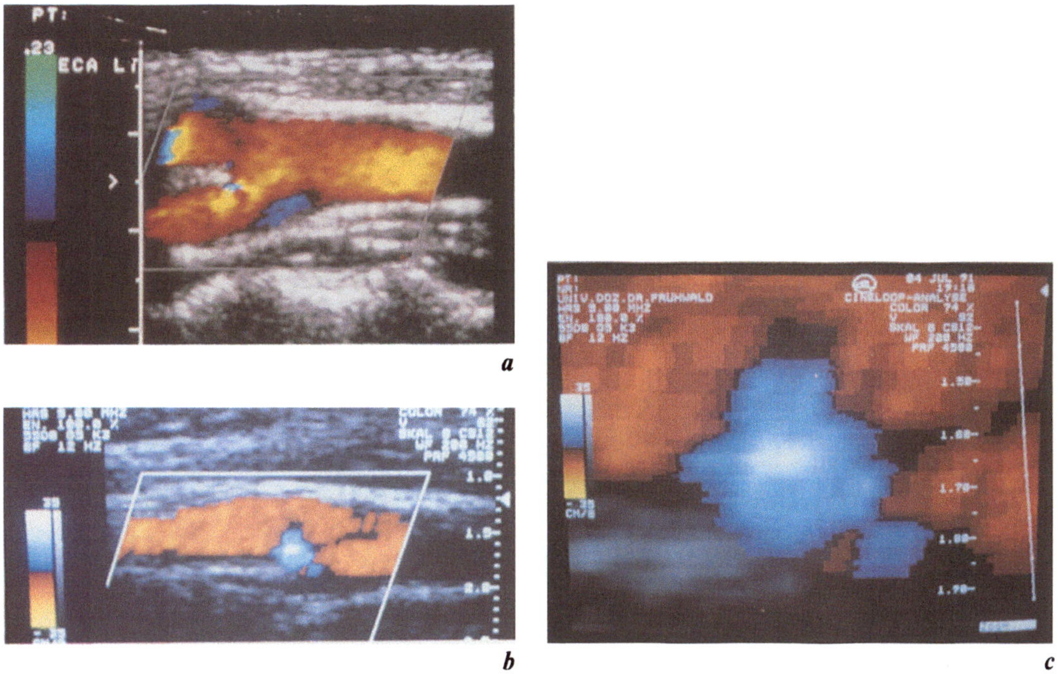

Fig. 7. ***a, b*** Physiologic flow separation seen in these normal carotid bulb images is easily differentiated from aliasing by the presence of black (indicating no flow) between red and blue, and by transition from red to blue in deeper shades of color ***c***. Greatly magnified view of the area of flow separation shown in ***b*** for better demonstration of the black border

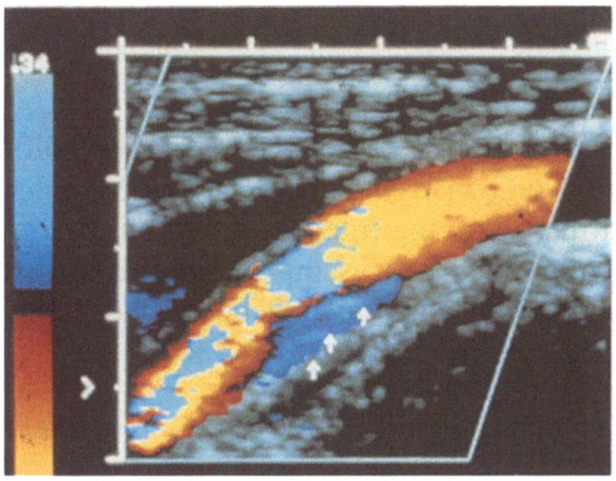

Fig. 8. Both flow separation (white arrows) and aliasing are shown in this single image of a normal carotid bulb; the aliasing is due to low Doppler angle values along the more distal portions of the vessel as it curves into the path of the beam

the least satisfactory approach to this problem since this technique also discards potentially important information about low flow values in diastole or in vessels with "slow flow". A better solution involves limiting low frequency values with high amplitude or applying algorithms which identify and selectively suppress typical tissue-movement patterns (Omoto, 1987; Taylor, 1990; Mitchell, 1990). Exclusion of color-coded pixels from areas already containing gray scale data has already been mentioned above. A smoother color display can also be obtained by

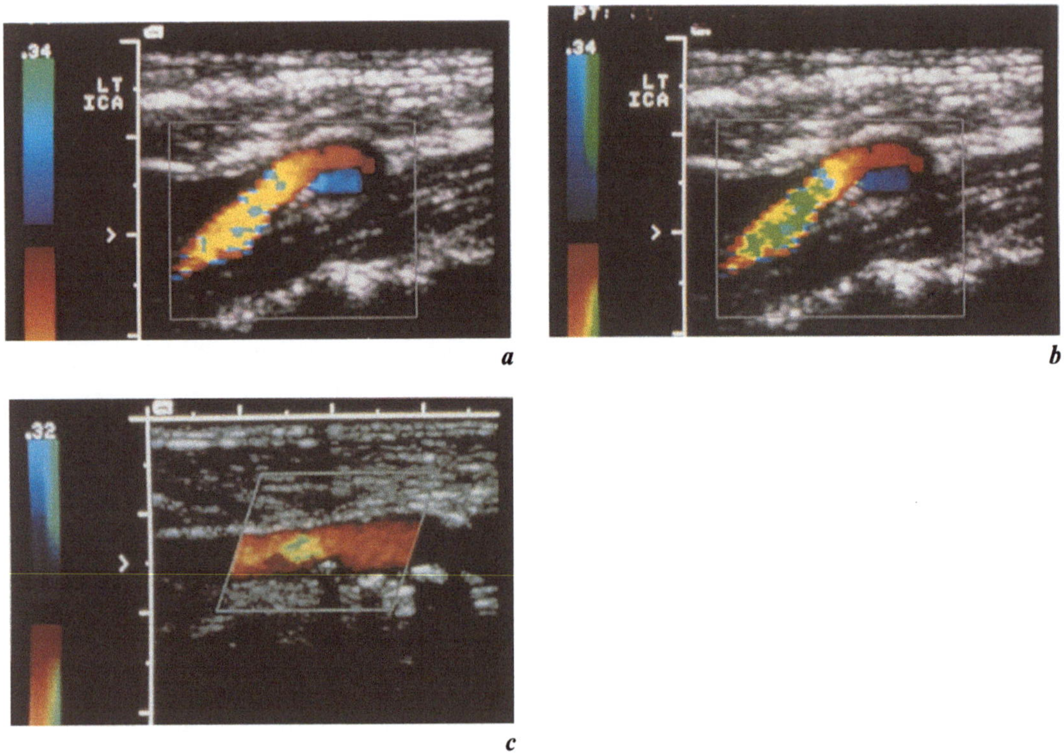

Fig. 9. Color encoding of turbulence: ***a*** Normal color map applied to area of turbulence; ***b*** Turbulence detection map (indicated by the split color bar at the left of the image) assigns green color to areas characterized by flow of both high and low velocities and various directions (turbulence); ***c*** Use of the turbulence detection map can be particularly helpful in identification of small regions of disturbed flow

use of spatial persistence techniques (filling the small gaps between adjacent color pixels), spatial filtering (displaying only those color pixels adjacent to other color pixels), or temporal persistence manipulations involving integration of data from several successive frames. The extent to which such processing techniques affect accurate depiction of complex hemodynamic events has not yet been extensively explored (Mitchell, 1990).

The future of CCDS

In the near future it is reasonable to expect continued improvement in design and performance of CCDS scanning instruments as computer speed and memory capabilities continue to increase in a cost-effective manner. This should eliminate the need for color line interpolation and allow higher true color line density at acceptable frame rates. Better algorithms for artifact recognition and suppression with minimal loss of useful data should also evolve. As the results of initial clinical studies of CCDS in various disease states become available, improvements in both scan technique and interpretation of findings can be expected.

New approaches to some existing limitations of CCDS can also be expected. At least one manufacturer is already addressing the issue of accurate *peak* velocity representation in the color display by providing a better match between angle calculation and the transducer elements within the array having the lowest angle of incidence relative to the direction of flow. Another company has taken a completely different approach to extracting flow information from the ultrasound data; this method is referred to as Color Velocity Imaging, or CVI. In CVI the *frequency* of the transducer is no longer a factor in the equation used for motion and velocity calculations. Smaller dwell time (ensemble length) requirements allow improved lateral resolution and full-frame color display without reduction in frame rate. Aliasing is not a problem with CVI, lower power output is required when compared to CCDS, and the color data can yield both *peak* velocity and volume flow information (Tegeler, 1991).

Advances in image storage, manipulation (such as correlation with previous scans), and transmission (for clinical availability or consultation) are certain to occur in the near future. It may become possible to integrate into a single display information acquired by ultrasound, CT, MRI and MR angiography, and EEG/biomagnetic modalities. This would have great potential for furthering the understanding of the relationship between seizure activity, masses, and vascular supply in the brain. Digital optical disk storage may become the archival method of choice as prices fall; this will facilitate recall of data with full measurement and calculation capability. Numeric values may be assigned to image features, facilitating identification of changes over a period of time or differences from one patient to another.

Further development of contrast agents for ultrasound may have a large impact on both vascular- and oncology-oriented color flow Doppler studies; "subtraction" imaging techniques may become available. Major innovation in display methods can be anticipated and may include 3-dimensional techniques, or even "virtual reality" displays which will allow the user to have the experience of being within an organ or vessel with ability to look in any direction; special gloves may allow tactile sensations to be provided and may help differentiate normal from abnormal parenchyma or determine the nature of plaque along vessel walls.

Acoustic holography may also find a niche in the diagnostic armamentarium although previous efforts have been limited by inconstant phase-change values in different tissues.

Undoubtedly, as in the past, the most exciting future developments are likely to be in areas which we cannot yet even imagine! Those of us fortunate enough to be involved in this discipline can only wait in eager anticipation of what lies ahead.

References

Atkinson P, Woodcock JP (1982) Doppler ultrasound and its use in clinical measurement. New York, Academic Press

Burns PN (1987) The physical principles of Doppler and spectral analysis. JCU 15: 567–590

Daigle R (1989) Quantitative aspects of color flow imaging. In: Nanda NC (ed) Textbook of color Doppler echocardiography. Philadelphia, Lea & Febiger, 283–291

Eden A (1990) Lecture: Doppler the man (revisited). Center for Medical Ultrasound of the Bowman Gray School of Medicine of Wake Forest University, February 16

Foley WD, Erickson SJ (1991) Color Doppler flow imaging. AJR 156: 3–13

Gessert JM, Moore GW (1987) Color flow imaging display modes and data acquisition parameters. Echocardiography 4: 375–381

Gill RW, Kossoff MB, Kossoff G, Griffiths KA (1989) New class of pulsed Doppler US ambiguity at short ranges. Radiology 173: 272–275

Hübsch P, Hager F, Benes E (1992) Color coded Doppler sonography of the male urethra during voiding: New observations of flow in an aqueous medium and their physical foundations. Frontiers in Europ Radiol Vol 9 (in press)
Kasai C (1989) Principles of Doppler color flow mapping. In: Nanda NC (ed) Textbook of color Doppler echocardiography. Philadelphia, Lea & Febiger, 14–17
Kremkau FW, Taylor KJW (1986) Artifacts in ultrasound imaging. J Ultrasound Med 5: 227–237
Klewer SE, Lloyd TR, Goldberg SJ (1989) In vivo relation between cineangiographic jet width and jet width imaged by color Doppler. Am J Cardiol 64:1399–1401
Lee R (1989) Physical principles of flow mapping in cardiology. In: Nanda NC (ed) Textbook of color Doppler echocardiography. Philadelphia, Lea & Febiger, 18–49
Merritt CRB (1991) Doppler US: The basics. Radiographics 11:109–119
Mitchell DG, Burns P, Needleman L (1990) Color Doppler artifact in anechoic regions. J Ultrasound Med 9: 255–260
Mitchell DG, Needleman L, Bezzi M et al (1987) Femoral artery pseudoaneurysm: Diagnosis with conventional duplex and color Doppler US. Radiology 165:687–690
Mitchell DG (1990) Color Doppler imaging: Principles, limitations, and artifacts. Radiology 177:1–10
Omoto R, Kasai C (1987) Physics and instrumentation of Doppler color flow mapping. Echocardiography 4:467–482
Powis RL (1983) Color flow imaging: Understanding its science and technology. J Diagn Med Sonography 4:236–245
Rubin JM (1991) Color Doppler image production. AIUM Color Doppler Sonography Symposium Syllabus, February 1991, Atlanta, Georgia
Stevenson JG (1989) Two-dimensional color Doppler estimation of the severity of atrioventricular valve regurgitation: important effects of instrument gain setting, pulse repetition frequency, and carrier frequency. J Am Soc Echocardiography 2:1–10
Taylor KJW, Holland S (1990) Doppler US, Part I: Basic principles, instrumentation, and pitfalls. Radiology 174:297–307
Tegeler CH, Kremkau FW, Hitchings LP (1991) Color velocity imaging: Introduction to a new ultrasound technology. J Neuroimag 1:85–90

2
CCDS: Optimizing instrument settings, scan techniques, and measurement procedures

D. E. Blackwell and F. Frühwald

The scanning environment

While a thorough understanding of the operating characteristics of any ultrasound scanning instrument has always been important for acquiring optimal images, even with gray-scale-only units, such an understanding becomes of critical importance with the additional features provided on duplex- and color-flow Doppler scanners. A few basic considerations with regard to the scanning environment deserve mention before we begin a more detailed look at how to optimize the various CCDS scan parameters. Comfort of both the sonographer and patient is an important factor, especially when a lengthy examination is anticipated; a restless patient or a shaky hand on the transducer can render a study useless even when state-of-the-art equipment is being used. If the patient is on a scanning table or stretcher (gurney) it is important that the mattress be sufficiently thick and firm to prevent uncomfortable pressure points; supplemental use of pillows under the knees or for partial elevation of the head (if allowed by the type of study to be performed) will contribute to the patient's ability to minimize movement. The sonographer should choose a position (whether standing or seated on an adjustable stool) which relieves rather than promotes strain. For carotid/vertebral artery studies some laboratories place the patient in an adjustable chair of the type used by dentists or barbers; the sonographer is seated behind the patient's head, and the back of the chair is reclined to bring the neck into easy reach. This approach is particularly appreciated by patients who have difficulty breathing when fully supine.

The console of the scanning instrument should also be where the sonographer can reach all the controls without straining; a supply of scanning gel and film should be close at hand and any foot controls (such as those used for freezing an image or exposing film) should be positioned for ease of access. Interior lighting in the scanning room should be controlled by a dimmer so that optimum balance of room light and display screen illumination can be obtained. Overhead light fixtures should not cause reflections from the imaging screens. Adequate soundproofing or isolation from noise is necessary if audible Doppler signal information is to be used for guidance and interpretation.

Choice of linear array, sector, or curved array transducers

The choice of a particular type of transducer for a given type of CCDS examination depends on the depth of the vessels of interest as well as their course relative to the skin surface. Decisions regarding the choice of frequency and focal characteristics are based in part on the usual trade-offs between resolution (better with higher frequencies) and penetration (better with lower frequencies). But when CCDS imaging is to be carried out, proper selection also requires an understanding of the beam geometry for each type of transducer. Linear phased array transducers, including those with electronic steering of the Doppler beam angle, present a constant angle of the beam to the skin surface and underlying structures (Fig. 1). This configuration is often the most useful for evaluation of the carotid and vertebral arteries as well as for upper and lower extremity vascular structures, thyroid and testicular scans, and breast imaging. Unidirectional flow in a vessel running roughly parallel to the skin surface will be color-coded in a single color throughout its course through the transducer's field of view.

Sector transducers, with their fan-shaped field of view, have a beam directed perpendicular to the skin and underlying structures centrally; the beam is angled away from the 90-degree central pattern on each side. The result of this is shown in Fig. 2; the same vessel pattern shown in a single color by the linear transducer now shows red-encoded flow on one end and blue-encoded flow on the other. Near 90 degrees no flow is registered (black). Close to the area imaged as black the colors are deeper (lower Doppler shift values because of near-90 degree angle of insonation). Clearly this type of display could cause confusion in interpreting the true flow characteristics of any underlying vessels. The properties of the sector scanner in CCDS can actually be used to advantage, however, when evaluating vascular structures with courses nearly perpendicular to the skin. It is likely that at least some portion of the vessel will be well displayed in the fan-shaped field of view, after which adjustments of instrument settings and transducer position can be carried out to optimize duplex Doppler cursor positioning and spectral analysis. Sector scanners of relatively low frequency are often used for abdominal and pelvic Doppler studies (renal, mesenteric, celiac, gynecologic).

Curved (phased) array transducers show beam geometry intermediate between the linear and sector patterns; the exact pattern will vary with the radius of curvature of the array (Fig. 3). The field of view near the transducer will be wider than with a sector transducer, but there will still be a change from red to blue color-coding for a vessel crossing the entire field of view (compare Fig. 2 and Fig. 3).

Electronic beam steering (as indicated by the parallelogram outlined in thin white lines in Fig. 1) can be used to improve an otherwise unsatisfactory Doppler insonation angle when actual physical repositioning of the scanhead is inadequate.

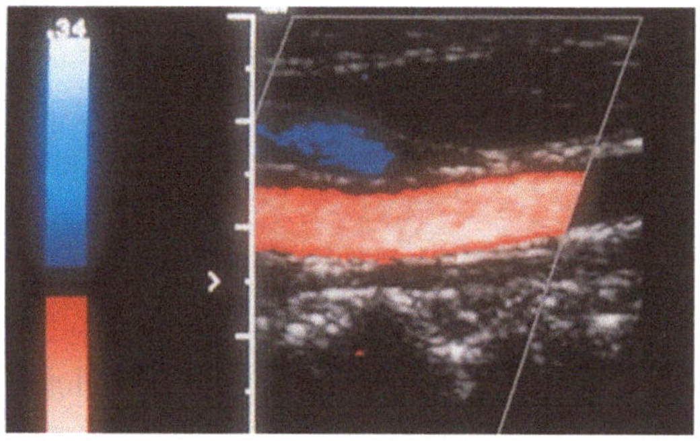

Fig. 1. Characteristic CCDS image obtained with a linear transducer: since there is a constant angle between the Doppler beam and the column of flowing blood, the entire vessel lumen is recorded in the same color (red in this case). Note the white parallelogram indicating an offset angle for the Doppler beam and defining the area of interest to be displayed in color

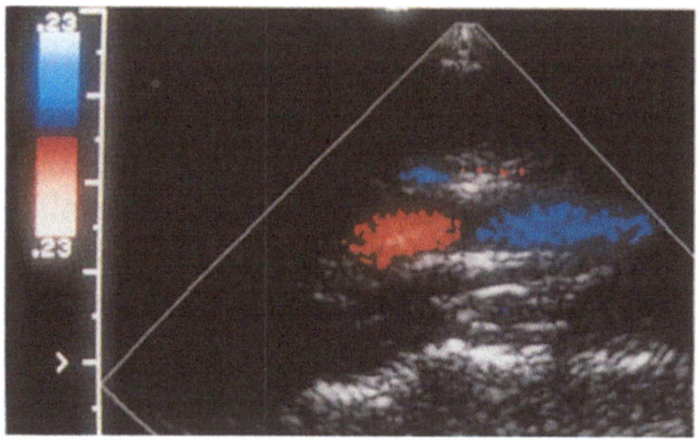

Fig. 2. Characteristic CCDS image obtained with a sector transducer: the angle of insonation reaches 90 degrees in the center of the image; flow to the right of center is displayed in blue and flow to the left of center in red (despite the fact that flow is actually unidirectional in this vessel)

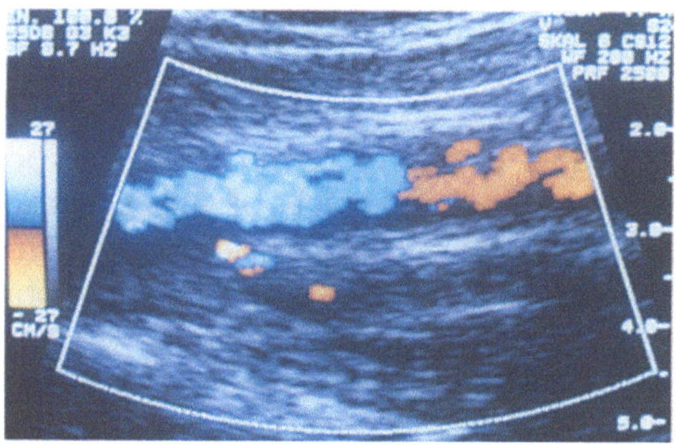

Fig. 3. This CCDS image obtained with a curved array transducer combines characteristics of both linear and sector transducers; there is a wider field of view close to the transducer than with a sector transducer but the problem of dual color assignment despite unidirectional flow is still present

As usual, there is a "trade-off" to consider: steering the beam at angles other than 90 degrees to the transducer surface decreases the effective aperture and increases the beam thickness. This can result in decreases in both sensitivity and lateral resolution and an increase in artifacts from grating lobes. Another approach to this beam-directing problem is to use a wedge-shaped block of material with acoustic properties similar to human tissue. When this is placed between the skin and transducer the entire array can be inclined to a new scan angle. Here the disadvantages are reverberation artifacts at the wedge-transducer and wedge-skin interfaces, increased attenuation, and increased transducer-to-target distance which may require reduced PRF values.

Proper use of CCDS set-up parameters

Successful use of CCDS instruments requires that the sonographer or physician operating the unit be fully comfortable with standard gray scale techniques and with details of the anatomy of the region to be evaluated. The operator must also be aware of the particular Doppler-oriented features present on his or her actual scanner. Many CCDS units provide several sets of stored parameters which can be used as initial settings for a particular type of examination such as carotid artery or deep (abdominal) vessel evaluation. Most scanners also offer the user the option of saving customized sets of parameters. These preset values, however, can only serve as a starting point for any given examination; careful adjustment of multiple system controls is necessary for maximizing the quality of each study. The guidelines provided below should prove useful to users of any of the CCDS units currently provided by major manufacturers, although the exact terminology applied to specific controls may vary. For example, most scanners will not have direct control over the pulse repetition frequency (PRF): to increase the PRF the operator should decrease the range setting on the Doppler scale; further increase in PRF can then be obtained by reducing the field of view (Middleton, 1991).

In most instances it is useful to obtain a good gray scale image of the body region of interest before enabling the color-flow overlay. Particular attention should be given to avoiding gray scale artifacts; a somewhat lower overall gain level than normally used may be appropriate, particularly on those scanners which will not color-encode areas where gray scale information has already been "written". Excessive gain resulting in artifactual echo patterns within the lumen of a vessel can lead to a false impression of luminal narrowing when color is excluded from the areas of gray scale artifact.

Careful attention should be given to the proper choice of power settings. Too little power may result in unsatisfactory color-coding of vessels of interest; too much power can cause excessive generation of artifacts. On some scanning instruments certain transducers automatically "default" to low power settings for obstetrical/fetal use. In some instances such transducers may not be satisfactory for peripheral vascular applications.

When the color circuitry is activated the color gain (and reject) controls should be set so that color "noise" is just visible and then reduced to just below the noise threshold. This setting will give optimum display of actual areas of flow. In some anatomic settings scanning of a vessel may produce a mirror image of the vessel (including its CCDS flow image). This occurs when some structure causing virtually 100% reflection of the ultrasound energy lies just beyond the target vessel. Lung filled with air can act as such a reflector and accounts for the well-recognized mirror image artifact of the right liver lobe as energy is reflected between the right lung base and the transducer. Similar reflection from lung at the apex and parasternal areas can result in duplication artifacts of the subclavian and internal mammary arteries (Middleton, 1991) (Fig. 5). If such mirror-image color flow artifacts are encountered they can often be minimized or eliminated by reduction in color gain, increase in color reject, or a combination of both. The same technique may help to minimize the "color mosaic" artifacts related to tissue vibration near a stenotic vessel or high-volume-flow dialysis shunt or A-V fistula.

As particular vascular patterns are identified it is important to optimize both the transducer position on the skin surface and the use of electronic Doppler angle correction (if available). In complete contrast to B-scan technique, where it is often desirable have the beam close to 90 degrees to a target's surface for maximum echo return, optimal CCDS flow imaging requires a Doppler angle in the 30 to 60 degree range if an accurate representation of flow velocity is to be obtained. This may require a physical shift in transducer position on the skin surface, an adjustment electronically to "steer" the Doppler beam in a more favorable direction, use of a tissue-equivalent "wedge", or (as is most often the case) some combination of these techniques.

Another choice to be made at this point concerns the area within the gray scale image to be designated for color display (usually referred to as the "area of interest" or "color field of view"). This must be large enough to provide the necessary "overview" of regional vessels but not so large as to cause excessive reduction in frame rate. Often it may be helpful to start with a fairly large area of interest and then reduce it to a "coned-in" view of particular target areas. The size of the area of interest is only one factor which affects frame rate. An increase in line density (which improves lateral resolution) will also cause a reduction in frame rate. Some instruments use interpolation of lines to increase apparent line density while maintaining the frame rate; this technique is acceptable when imaging large vessels but may result in loss of important data when vessels of small diameter are evaluated. Settings optimal for detection of "slow flow" require a slower pulse repetition frequency (PRF) and longer "dwell time" (the duration of Doppler sampling for each line of sight; increasing the dwell time improves Doppler accuracy); both of these factors result in reduced frame rate. Trade-offs must then be consciously made depending on the particular vascular structures being interrogated. In cardiac applications where large areas of high-velocity flow are typical, high frame rates can be used since temporal resolution is more important than spatial resolution. The converse is generally true for abdominal and peripheral vascular applications, where the detection of relatively slow flow or the resolution of small vessels is the goal and lower frame rates required.

Slow flow must be detected for effective CCDS imaging of small arteries and most veins. Erythrocytes act as point scatterers of ultrasound; the combined effect of such reflection is referred to as *Rayleigh-Tyndall scattering*. For target elements in this size range the intensity of the scattered wave increases with the fourth power of the transducer frequency; doubling the frequency value results in a sixteen-fold increase in returning echo intensity (Burns, 1991). It is therefore easy to see why it becomes important to choose the highest frequency transducer compatible with necessary penetration to the depth of the vessels to be evaluated. Wall filter settings should be minimized to avoid loss of low-frequency Doppler shift information. It may be necessary to decrease the PRF and increase the dwell time settings to maximize sensitivity to slow flow. These instrument settings tend to make the scanner quite sensitive to transducer and tissue motion; slow, deliberate positioning of the scanhead will help to minimize motion ("color flash") artifacts.

Aliasing

In addition to mirror image (Fig. 5), tissue vibration, and color flash artifacts there is at least one more important CCDS artifact which must be understood; this is referred to as aliasing. Accurate (mean) flow velocity representation by CCDS becomes impossible when returning Doppler shift values exceed one half of the pulse repetition frequency (a value referred to as the *Nyquist limit*). When the Nyquist limit is exceeded for a vessel being displayed in red, there will be an abrupt change from *light* shades of red to *light* shades of blue, often centrally within the vessel where flow velocities tend to be the highest in the presence of a normal laminar flow pattern (see Fig. 16 in Carotid Artery chapter). In cases where *actual* reversal of flow direction occurs the change from red to blue will occur in the darker shades of color, as flow slows prior to changing direction. Physicians and sonographers who have worked with duplex Doppler and spectral analysis of Doppler waveform patterns will be familiar with the same artifact, which appears as a "clipped" peak of a Doppler wave pattern which is then displayed on the opposite side of the baseline (see Fig. 15 in Carotid Artery chapter).

In CCDS studies, recognition of aliasing is often a useful clue to the location of areas of highest flow velocity, such as points of maximal carotid artery, dialysis shunt, or A-V fistula flow acceleration. Once such an area is identified then sample volume placement for spectral analysis can be readily accomplished. If aliasing is also encountered in the spectral waveform display it may be necessary to use higher PRF values, a Doppler angle closer to 90 degrees (remembering that angles greater than 60 degrees are associated with decreasing accuracy of measurement), or a transducer of lower frequency (or even a continuous-wave Doppler instrument in some settings, since CW units are not subject to aliasing).

Measurement techniques

While fairly extensive coverage has been given in the Carotid Artery chapter to proper measurement techniques for determining the degree of vessel stenosis, a few points deserve particular emphasis. In order to be as accurate as possible when residual luminal area is to be determined it is important that adequate "slow-flow" sensitivity be used so that even the layer of blood with sluggish flow near the vessel wall (or adjacent to an area of plaque or thrombus formation) will be color-encoded. If such slow-flow areas are excluded due to improper settings, then an overestimation of the degree of stenosis may be made. With this precaution in mind, a long-axis scan through the area of maximal narrowing is obtained (Fig. 4a). The transducer is then rotated 90 degrees and a transverse image through the area of maximal stenosis is obtained. Slight cephalad (or rarely, caudad) angulation relative to the true cross sectional plane is desirable since flow detection will be facilitated by a more optimal angle of insonation. While this may produce a somewhat more elliptical cross-sectional image of the vessel, the effect on the final measurements is negligible. The perimeter of the entire vessel is marked (Fig. 4b) and the area computed; the perimeter of the color-coded residual lumen is then similarly marked (Fig. 4c), its area calculated, and the ratio of its area to the area of the entire vessel is computed. Percent area stenosis is then defined as $(1 - \text{residual lumen area}/\text{vessel lumen area}) \times 100$.

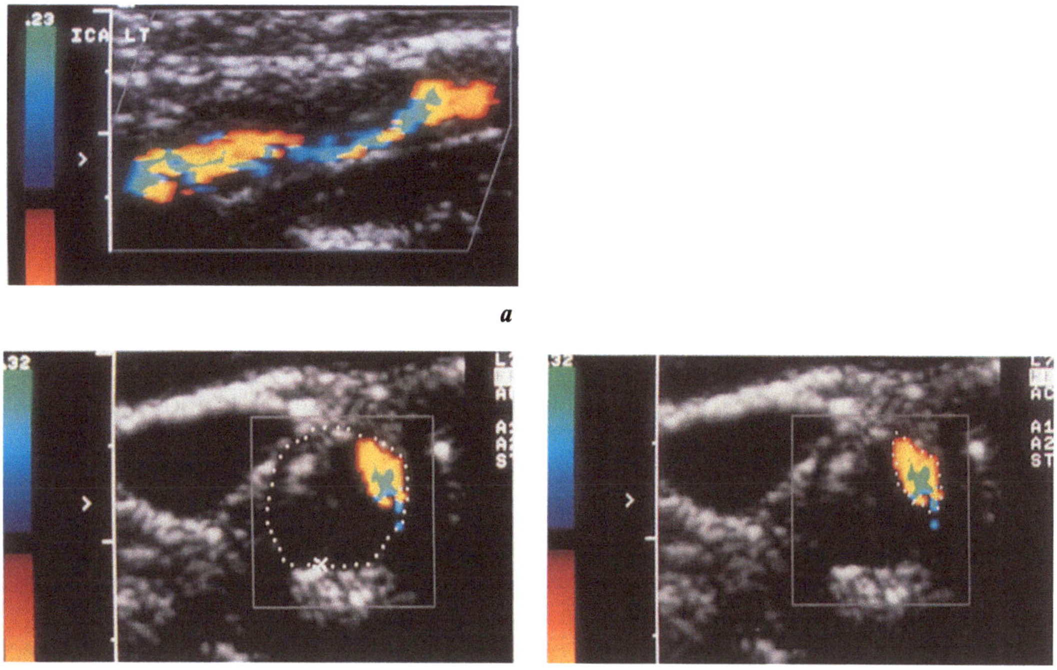

a

b *c*

Fig. 4. ***a*** Longitudinal scan of a high-grade stenosis of a proximal ICA. Percent area stenosis measurement is carried out in transverse images with tracing of the circumference of the entire vessel wall ***b*** and then similar measurement of the residual lumen ***c***

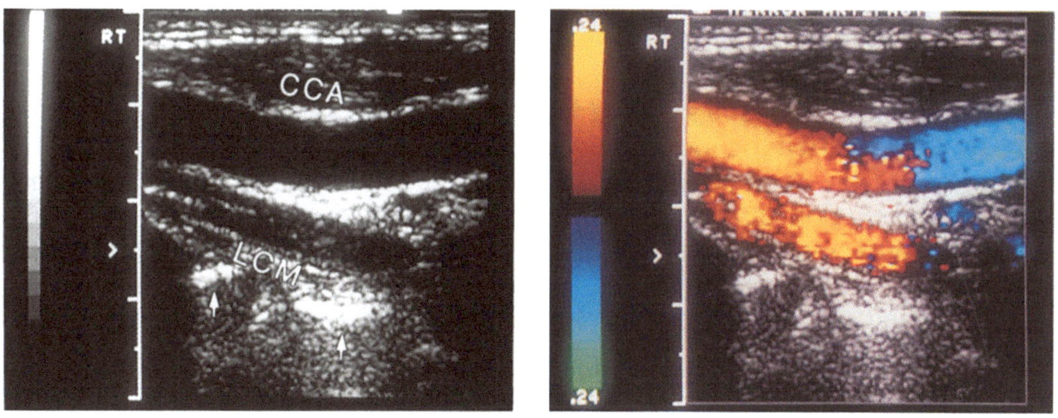

a *b*

Fig. 5. Mirror image artifact of the common carotid artery: ***a*** Common carotid artery (CCA) and longus colli muscle (LCM) on a gray scale picture. (Cervical vertebral bodies: arrows) In color mode there is a mirror artifact from the CCA on the LCM ***b***

As noted in the section on aliasing, the color flow image cannot be used for accurate assessment of *peak* flow velocity since in most scanners each color pixel represents a *mean* flow value. While technical approaches to accurate peak velocity display directly from the color Doppler screen are being evaluated for the next generation of CCDS units, accurate measurement currently requires spectral analysis; CCDS, however, greatly facilitates precise positioning of the sample volume for acquisition of spectral waveform data. In cases where calcified plaque causes acoustic shadowing of the lumen, neither CCDS nor spectral analysis can directly obtain accurate data concerning the degree of underlying stenosis. Careful evaluation of flow information available proximal and distal to the area of shadowing can often give important clues as to the severity of stenosis in the obscured segment, however.

Appendix I gives the formulas for several of the most commonly used indices for spectral waveform analysis. The resistance index (RI) is useful in detection of an increase in peripheral resistance as may be encountered in the extracranial ICA when stenosis is present distally in the intracranial portion of the vessel. Another indicator of increased distal resistance is a prolonged *acceleration time* (AT), obtained by measuring the time between the diastolic minimum and the systolic maximum. The pulsatility index (PI) increases as the difference between peak systolic and diastolic frequency (or velocity) becomes greater; note that this index requires the *mean* velocity in the denominator. The A/B ratio simply consists of the peak systolic value divided by the peak diastolic value and has been extensively used in obstetrical umbilical vessel evaluation; it is limited to some extent by the fact that zero diastolic values result in a value of infinity.

In cases of carotid stenosis our preferred measurement approach is direct measurement of percent area stenosis from the transverse CCDS images as described above. If this is not technically satisfactory or if intracranial ICA stenosis is suspected, then careful attention is given to RI, AT, and ICA/CCA ratio (see table at end of Carotid chapter) values. If these are abnormal then we recommend further investigation using transcranial Doppler, magnetic resonance imaging, magnetic resonance angiography, or conventional angiography depending on the clinical presentation of the patient.

It is very important to be aware that no single measurement considered in isolation from other findings should be relied upon for determining the degree of stenosis. Careful attention must be given to direct measurement, use of indices, and comparison of the contralateral vessels. A severe ICA stenosis or occlusion may lead to increased flow through the contralateral carotid system; this can give a false impression of stenosis (or a more severe degree of stenosis). Absolute measurement values vary widely depending upon the patient's blood pressure, cardiac status, heart rate, and other factors; relative measurements such as the ICA/CCA ratio help to minimize the effect of such variables.

A few words should be said about measurement in non-carotid CCDS studies. As pointed out in the chapter on Dialysis Fistula evaluation, some attempts have been made to quantitate flow volume through the shunt, not only to determine adequacy of flow for dialysis but to identify cases in which excessive flow may be contributing to cardiac compromise or other problems (Oates, 1990). Appendix II gives the formula for volume flow calculation and a short computer program which has in our experience often provided a useful approximation of flow volume even when the numeric average of peak systolic and diastolic flow velocity values is substituted for the true time-averaged mean flow velocity. Flow volume values are calculated for both the arterial and venous limbs of the fistula; it is normal for the venous segment to have somewhat lower values since the feeding artery may also be contributing flow to some arterial tributaries. The 1990 article by Oates et al. gives a good overview of the advantages and limitations of flow volume calculation from Doppler parameters.

Finally, in the evaluation of venous compromise due to thrombosis, compression, or tumor invasion it is important to look at such parameters as flow changes with respiration and Valsalva (absence of changes suggests flow through a narrowed venous lumen or through small collateral veins) and response to augmentation and compression maneuvers. Direct observation of the patient should also not be overlooked; edema of a limb, distension of neck veins, and coloration changes in the skin are all important clues to the status of underlying vascular structures. In evaluation of upper extremity and thoracic outlet arteries, careful documentation of bilateral brachial blood pressure values is essential to proper interpretation of CCDS and spectral analysis findings. A detailed vascular history (muscle fatigue or pain, intermittent swelling, diabetes mellitus, hypertension, coronary artery disease, recent or remote trauma to an extremity, etc.) should also never be overlooked since it can often help "focus" the examination.

Image storage techniques

Most recent CCDS instruments will have the ability to capture and store (in digital memory) the last several seconds of the examination as it proceeds. This sequence of scan images can be reviewed to allow selection of precisely the desired frames for long-term storage. A videorecorder is one commonly used method of archiving examinations; high-quality images with good color purity are essential for accurate review and interpretation of CCDS examinations, and one of the newer high-resolution formats such as S-VHS or Hi-8 mm should be used. Some instruments now allow information from tape to be played back into digital memory so that measurement calipers and other tools can be used just as during an actual scan. The ability to produce an accurate freeze-frame image from tape is also important and will most often be accomplished by the use of a digital memory frame-buffer for stable display. Color hard-copy images can be obtained with an instant-film color camera, thermal-transfer color printer, color slide recorder, or color laser imager (the latter being the latest and most expensive option).

Quality control and standardization

As with all ultrasound scanning instruments, a program of ongoing quality control is essential for CCDS units. Many manufacturers provide detailed information on each transducer shipped with the scanner, including power output values, beam geometry, and other parameters. This information is very helpful in re-evaluation of a transducer if its performance seems to be degraded, or in a regular schedule of quality control checks. It is also helpful to obtain images of a tissue-equivalent phantom at standardized power and sensitivity settings whenever a new transducer is placed in service so that comparison images can be made as needed. These measures can be carried out as a part of the manufacturer-provided series of preventive maintenance service visits or as an "in-house" quality control activity. Several ultrasound phantoms are now available which include some mechanism for checking the accuracy of Doppler flow-velocity values; these devices incorporate a calibrated moving target such as a motor-driven string or pump-and-tubing system. These phantoms can be useful in training programs, where the effects of transducer positioning and angulation can be easily appreciated, as well as in quality control and standardization activities.

Appendix I: Commonly used Doppler measurement indices

Resistance Index: (A – B)/A
Pulsatility Index: (A – B)/Mean
Systolic-Diastolic Ratio: A/B

Where A = Maximum Doppler shift frequency (or velocity) value in one cardiac cycle
B = Minimum Doppler shift frequency (or velocity) value in one cardiac cycle
Mean = The time-average of the maximum Doppler shift frequency (or velocity) value over the cardiac cycle (Burns, 1988)

Note that since these indices are *ratios* they are not angle-dependent and can be applied even to vessels too small or tortuous for accurate assessment of the Doppler angle, or in cases where Doppler angles greater than 60 degrees must be used (Burns, 1988).

Appendix II: Formula for flow volume estimation

$VO = V \times A \times 60$ seconds

Where VO = Flow volume in cubic centimeters per minute
V = Mean flow velocity in cm/sec
A = Vessel lumen area in square centimeters

If mean flow velocity is not calculated and displayed by your particular scanning unit a workable approximation can be obtained using the formula $V = D + ((S - D)/2)$, where D = peak diastolic flow velocity in cm/sec and S = peak systolic flow velocity in cm/sec, and V = Average of systolic and diastolic peak flow velocity values.

The following is a short computer program in BASIC which allows rapid calculation of shunt flow volume values:

```
10 REM FISTFLOW.BAS – A program to calculate volume flow
90 CLS
100 INPUT "VESSEL AREA IN SQUARE CM (OR 0 TO USE DIAMETERS):
";A
110 IF A>0 THEN 240
200 INPUT "VESSEL DIAMETER #1 IN CM: ";D1
220 INPUT "VESSEL DIAMETER #2 IN CM: ";D2
240 INPUT "PEAK SYSTOLIC VELOCITY IN CM/SEC: ";S
260 INPUT "PEAK DIASTOLIC VELOCITY IN CM/SEC: ";D
300 PRINT" "
390 IF A>0 THEN 440
400 R=(D1+D2)/4
420 A=(R*R)*3.1416
440 V=D+((S-D)/2)
500 VO=V*A*60
510 PRINT "FLOW VOLUME ESTIMATE IS ";:PRINT USING
"#####";VO;:PRINT" CC/MIN"
520 PRINT" (ACCURACY IS PROBABLY NO BETTER THAN +/- 25%)"
```

References

Burns PN (1988) Interpretation and analysis of Doppler signals. Chapter 4. In: Taylor KJW, Burns PN, Wells PNT (eds) Clinical applications of Doppler ultrasound. New York, Raven Press

Burns PN (1991) Basic Doppler principles. From the Syllabus of the advanced color Doppler ultrasonography course, American Institute of Ultrasound in Medicine, Rockville, MD

Doppler Sonographic Imaging of the Vascular System (1991) Report of the Ultrasonography Task Force, Council on Scientific Affairs, American Medical Association. JAMA 265:2382–2387

Foley DW, Erickson SJ (1991) Color Doppler flow imaging. AJR 156:3–13

Medical Diagnostic Ultrasound Instrumentation and Clinical Interpretation (1991) Report of the Ultrasonography Task Force, Council on Scientific Affairs, American Medical Association. JAMA 265:1155–1159

Merritt CRB (1991) Doppler US: The basics. Radiographics 11:109–119

Middleton WD (1991) Color Doppler ultrasonography: Image interpretation and optimization. From the Syllabus of the Advanced Color Doppler Ultrasonography Course, American Institute of Ultrasound in Medicine, Rockville, MD

Middleton WD, Erickson S, Melson GL (1989) Perivascular color artifact: pathologic significance and appearance on color Doppler US images. Radiology 171(3):647–652

Middleton WD, Melson GL (1990) The carotid ghost. A color Doppler ultrasound duplication artifact. J Ultrasound Med 9(9):487–493

Mitchell DG (1990) Color Doppler imaging: Principles, limitations, and artifacts. Radiology 177: 1–10

Mitchell DG, Burns P, Needleman L (1990) Color Doppler artifact in anechoic regions. J Ultrasound Med 9(5):255–260

Oates CP, Williams ED, McHugh MI (1990) The use of a duplex ultrasound scanner to measure volume flow in arterio-venous fistulae in patients undergoing haemodialysis: an analysis of measurement uncertainties. Ultrasound Med Biol 16:571–579

Scoutt LM, Zawin ML, Taylor KJW (1990) Doppler US: Part II. Clinical applications. Radiology 174:309–319

Taylor KJW, Holland S (1990) Doppler US: Part I. Basic principles, instrumentation, and pitfalls. Radiology 174:297–307

The Future of Ultrasonography (1991) Report of the Ultrasonography Task Force, Council on Scientific Affairs, American Medical Association. JAMA 266:406–409

3
Color-coded Doppler sonography of the carotid arteries

S. Trattnig and P. Hübsch

Introduction

The relationship between extracranial carotid atherosclerosis, transient ischemic attacks and cerebral infarction is similar to that between coronary atherosclerosis and angina pectoris, myocardial infarction and sudden death. The prevalence of internal carotid artery (ICA) stenosis of any degree in subjects devoid of any cerebrovascular symptoms or signs is low in both sexes prior to 65 years of age. It is only 2.4% in males between the ages of 55 and 64 years, but it increases sharply with age, reaching 30.3% for stenosis of less than 50% and 6.1% for stenosis greater than 50% in males aged 75–84 years. The prevalence of minimal lesions (plaques causing less than 15% diameter reduction) is high: 32.1% in males aged 45–54 years and 48.5% in the 75 to 84 year age range. In all studies age is the most important risk factor for carotid atherosclerosis. Hypertension, diabetes mellitus, cigarette smoking and hyperlipidemia have also been associated with increased risk for cerebrovascular atherosclerosis. A recent study (Niederkorn, 1991) found a significant association between fibrinogen levels (as well as age) and the presence of carotid stenosis in a group of 125 asymptomatic subjects. Earlier studies had established a significant correlation between fibrinogen levels and *symptomatic* carotid artery disease (Lechner, 1987). It has been suggested that elevated fibrinogen may be an independent risk factor for stroke and may have value as a simple screening test to help establish the probability of early atherosclerotic carotid artery disease in asymptomatic patients even in the absence of other classic risk factors (Wilhelmson, 1984). *Progression* of stenosis (mean follow-up interval 26 months) was associated in Niederkorn's 1991 report with lower HDL cholesterol levels (average 44.5±13 mg/dl) than in subjects showing no interval increase in vessel narrowing (average values 57.9±18 mg/dl).

Carotid sonography using continuous-wave (CW) and duplex Doppler techniques has proven to be highly accurate in detecting and quantifying carotid atherosclerosis. By far the most common indication for these examinations is for triage of patients at risk for stroke. In the absence of significant stenosis, surgery is usually not considered. An abnormal ultrasound study, on the other hand, may lead to angiography and possibly endarterectomy.

The purpose of this chapter is to describe the advantages of color-coded Doppler sonography (CCDS) in the noninvasive evaluation of extracranial carotid artery disease in comparison to conventional sonography and the traditional "gold standard", angiography.

Examination technique

CCDS allows simultaneous display of a gray scale tissue image (B-mode) and superimposed color-coded Doppler information. Patients should be examined in the supine position with the head hyperextended and the neck either straight or obliqued in the contralateral direction. Since the carotid vessels are relatively superficial, a high frequency imaging probe (7.5–10 MHz) should be used to allow optimal visualization of vessel anatomy and vascular pathology in both transverse and sagittal planes (Figs. 1, 2). The proximal external carotid artery (ECA) is anteromedial to the ICA in approximately 95% of cases; in 5% it is posterolateral (Fig. 3). Usually, the ICA runs parallel to the jugular vein (Fig. 4). Color flow imaging allows differentiation of the carotid branches by demonstration of increased pulsatility in the ECA compared to the ICA in real-time; this can be nicely shown in the transverse plane. In most cases better differentiation of one or more branches of the ECA can be accomplished with CCDS than with non-color duplex scanning; this helps to avoid error in distinguishing the ICA and ECA, particularly in cases where obstructive disease is present (Fig. 5).

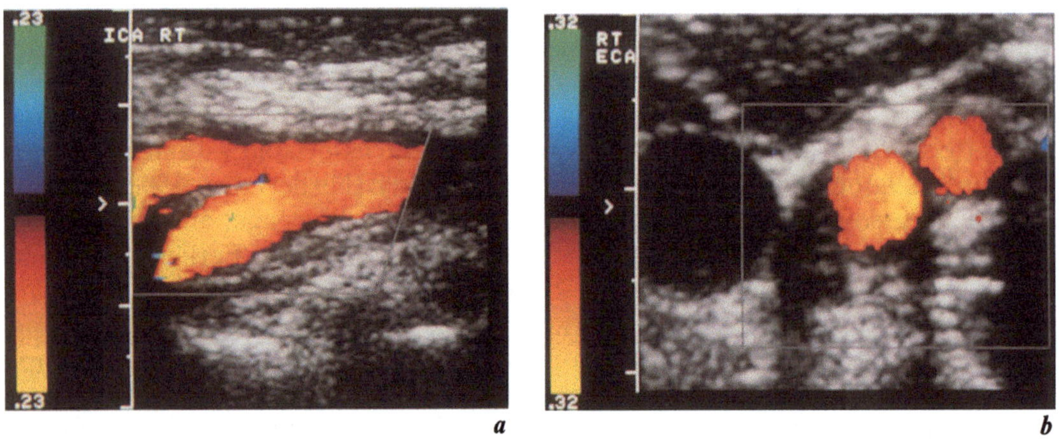

Fig. 1. ***a, b*** CCDS of carotid arteries in longitudinal and transverse plane: normal color-flow examination of CCA, carotid bifurcation and proximal portions of ICA and ECA in longitudinal plane

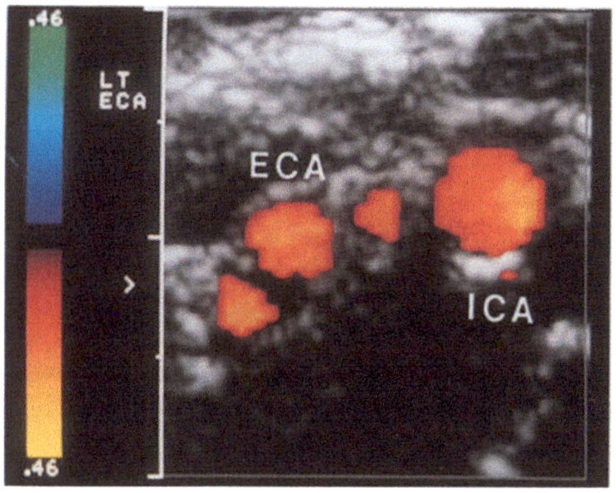

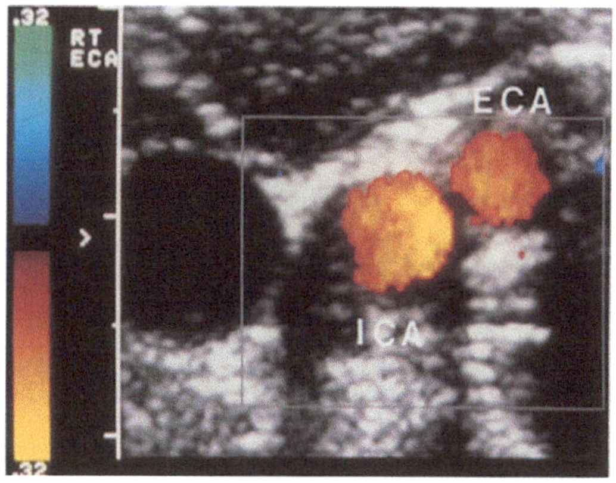

Fig. 2. (left) Good CCDS demonstration of ICA and ECA above the bifurcation including demonstration of two ECA branches

Fig. 3. (right) Transverse sonogram above the bifurcation: ECA runs anteromedial to ICA (in 95% of cases)

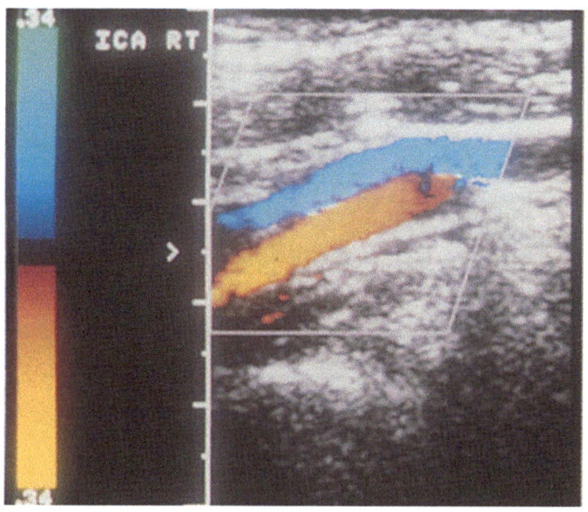

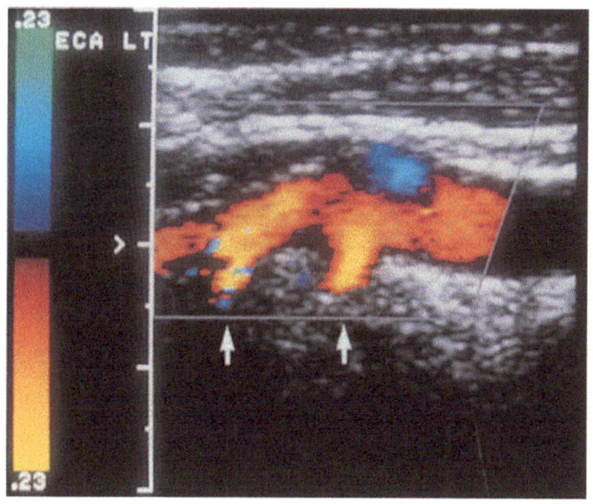

Fig. 4. (left) Longitudinal sonogram: ICA (red) runs parallel to the internal jugular vein (blue, because of opposite flow direction)

Fig. 5. (right) ECA in a longitudinal view with demonstration of two branches (superior thyroid artery and ascending pharyngeal artery: arrows)

The examination is carried out in two steps: first, multiple longitudinal and transverse B-mode images are obtained for determination of vessel course, detection of wall thickening and atheromatous lesions, and definition of plaque extent and morphology; next, color-coded blood flow is superimposed for evaluation of hemodynamics in general and for detailed analysis of any areas of pathology. Atheromatous plaques are analyzed for surface characteristics and structure, with the former being facilitated by observation of the presence or absence of color at each point along the contour of a suspected lesion. Color flow imaging is interpreted as normal if the lumen is homogeneously and completely color-coded with demonstration of a laminar flow pattern (higher flow velocities with less color saturation in the lumen center and lower velocities with deeper color saturation toward the vessel walls).

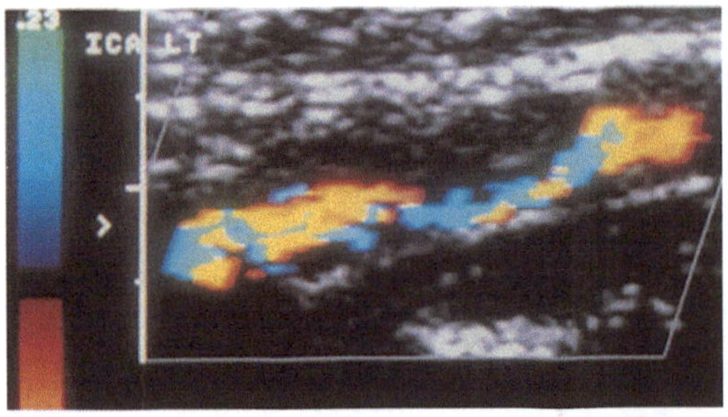

Fig. 6. CCDS demonstrates a jet of high-velocity flow that does not follow the long axis of the vessel. Because CCDS displays the true axis of blood flow in a vessel, it is useful in accurate Doppler angle correction

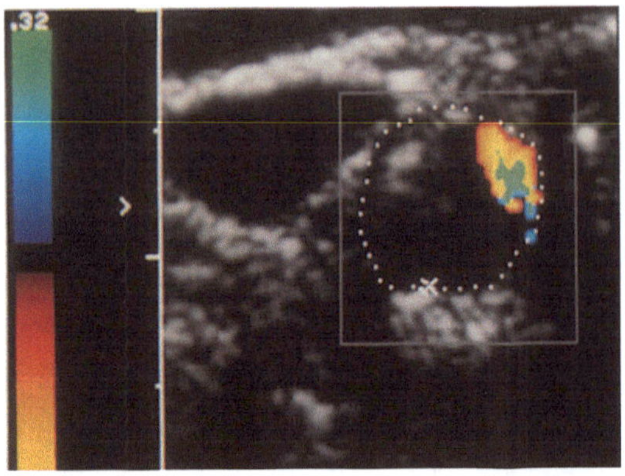

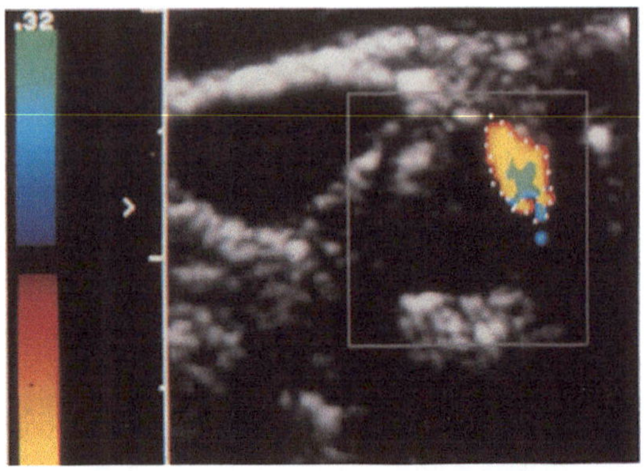

Figs. 7 (left), 8 (right). These transverse scans through the proximal ICA demonstrate the method for percent area stenosis measurement, with determination of circumferential measurement of the vessel wall and corresponding measurement of the residual lumen

Flow direction with respect to the transducer determines whether red or blue will be assigned to the color flow "map". At our institutions we use instrument settings which display flow toward the brain in red (normal carotid and vertebral artery pattern) and flow toward the chest in blue (cervical veins). For each examination the velocity color scale is adjusted to give as complete color encoding of the flow lumen as possible without causing aliasing (seen as a blue "island" within the red-encoded flow lumen). The sensitivity of the system for the detection of motion is set individually for each patient slightly above the level of color noise and is then reduced to just below the noise threshold. Stenoses with greater than 40% lumen narrowing are graded according to degree, extent and duration of reduced color saturation of the color-coded Doppler signal indicating high flow velocities, and the presence and characteristics of post-stenotic flow patterns. Peak systolic and end-diastolic flow velocities are routinely measured in the common carotid artery (CCA) one cm below the bifurcation, and in the proximal ICA and ECA. In cases of stenosis these flow velocities are recorded by placing the sample volume within the blood stream or flow jet, both within and immediately beyond the region of maximum stenosis. Angle correction is performed parallel to the residual color-coded lumen (Fig. 6). Direct measurement to determine the degree of stenosis is performed in the transverse plane. The area of the residual lumen of the ICA (as depicted in color) is divided into the total area of the vessel at the same level (Figs. 7, 8). For transverse-plane images a slight transducer tilt to provide a Doppler angle for simultaneous color Doppler display is necessary. Careful attention is given to differentiating normal blood flow from flow separation and flow reversal zones in the region of the carotid bifurcation. In patients with a high location of the bifurcation or inability to hyperextend the neck, the visualization of the carotid bifurcation is often facilitated by the use of a posterolateral approach with the internal jugular vein imaged in front of the carotid artery. In cases where the carotid system is quite deep in the neck better assessment may be obtained with a 5 MHz transducer.

Normal and abnormal hemodynamics in the extracranial carotid system

Numerous experimental studies have focused on the pattern of blood flow in the human carotid bifurcation. Glass models of the bifurcation and actual cadaver specimens have been used, and both pulsatile and non-pulsatile flow have been utilized to simulate the anatomic and physiologic conditions in vivo. These experiments have shown that there is an area of boundary layer separation where normal laminar flow is disrupted in conjunction with reversal of flow at the bifurcation, opposite the origin of the external carotid artery (Fig. 9). As blood passes through the lumen of an artery the frictional forces exerted by the wall surface retard the flow velocities in the adjacent layer. This laminar flow pattern can be demonstrated easily by CCDS with lower color saturation (lighter color shade) in the center of the vessel, indicating faster flowing blood in the center of the stream, and higher color saturation (deeper color shade) adjacent to the vessel wall representing lower flow velocities (Fig. 10). The region in which these forces are active is defined as a boundary layer. Fluid elements at a distance from the surface and outside the boundary layer are not affected by these viscous forces. Changes in geometry of the artery can result in blood moving against a pressure gradient, from low to high pressure regions, due to momentum. Blood with relatively low momentum, such as that within a boundary layer, may become stationary or may reverse flow direction. Thus an area of flow separation results and local regions of stagnant and reversed flow can develop (drawing 1). Some work has been done documenting flow reversal in vivo by means of duplex Doppler US and angiography, but a detailed analysis of the flow patterns in vivo has not previously been possible because of the lack of an appropriate imaging device. It is possible to document these flow components now that advances in technology allow real-time display of color-coded flow images (Fig. 11).

When atherosclerosis develops, it preferentially involves the posterolateral bulb region, obliterating the normal configuration of the sinus with resultant loss of the flow separation zone (Fig. 12). It has therefore been hypothesized that if flow separation can be detected, it should be predictive of a normal angiogram. The predilection of atheromatous lesions to form at certain sites in the arterial tree has long been noted. Atheroma occur principally at curves and the origins of branch vessels, where boundary layer separation occurs. It has been postulated that areas

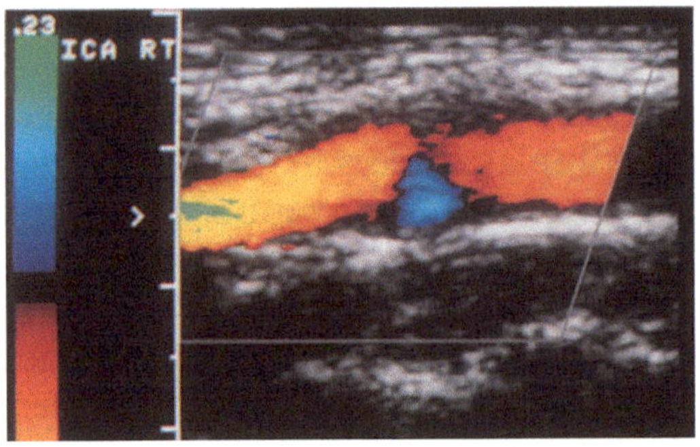

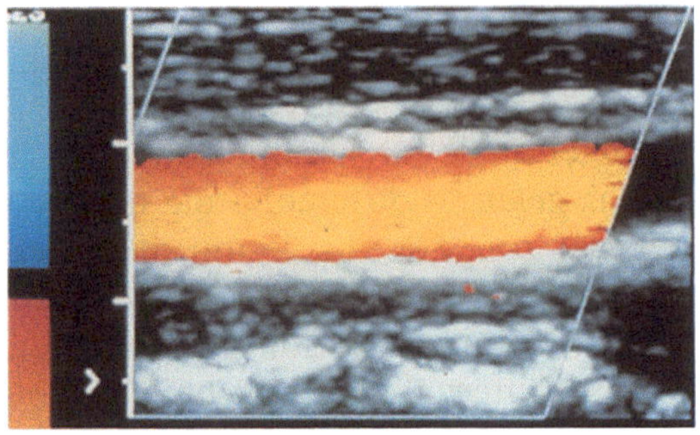

Fig. 9. (left) Longitudinal view of carotid artery bifurcation with flow reversal in the posterolateral region of the bifurcation shown as a blue "island" within the red blood stream

Fig. 10. (right) Longitudinal sonogram at mid-CCA level shows lower color saturation (lighter shade of color) in the center of the vessel and higher color saturation (deeper shade of color) adjacent to both vessel walls. This appearance is due to laminar flow with more rapidly flowing blood in the center of the stream

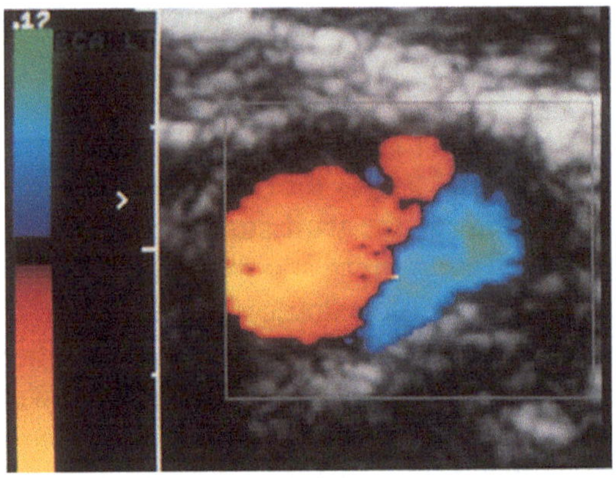

Fig. 11. Marked flow reversal at the carotid bifurcation in transverse plane

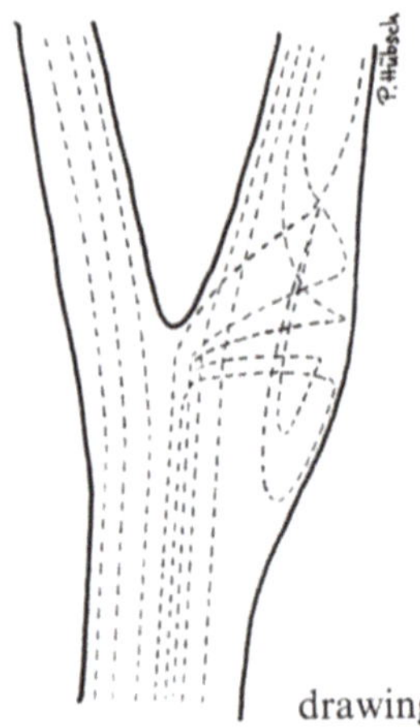

drawing 1

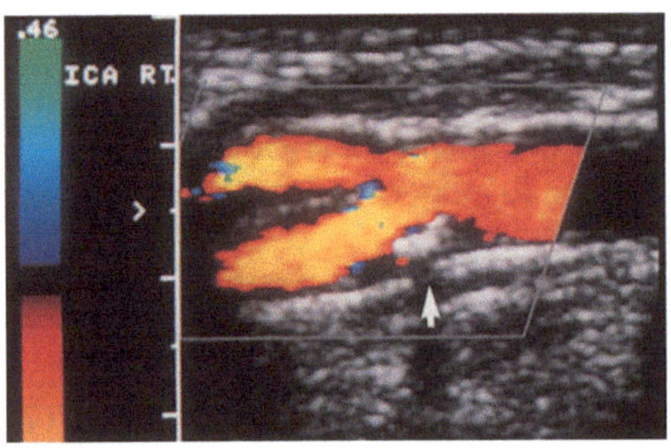

Fig. 12. Carotid bifurcation in a longitudinal view shows obliteration of normal configuration of the carotid sinus due to small atherosclerotic plaques on the posterior wall with resulting loss of a flow reversal zone (arrow)

of stasis occurring in regions of flow separation permit the aggregation and interaction of blood components, resulting in local plaque formation. The region of predicted flow reversal and boundary layer separation is easily confirmed with CCDS in healthy subjects. The dominant configuration appears to consist of peripheral flow reversal located opposite the origin of the external carotid artery and just below the bifurcation. Beyond the bifurcation the region of flow reversal may migrate to the center of the internal carotid artery and may assume either a continuous or an interrupted linear configuration, extending from the superficial to the deep wall of the internal carotid artery. However, several variations of this flow pattern have been described. In addition to the variability in configuration, there is also a great deal of variability in magnitude and duration of flow reversal (Figs. 13, 14). Therefore it is difficult to attach any significance to particular flow patterns in asymptomatic individuals. Perhaps long-term follow-up studies will determine if any particular flow pattern places an individual at risk for the development of focal atherosclerotic disease. The inability to separate normal from abnormal flow conditions induced by carotid plaques has been a major problem for conventional sonographic techniques. In CCDS it is important to distinguish between flow reversal zones and aliasing, which may both appear as a blue area within the red-encoded blood stream. Aliasing in a duplex spectral tracing is seen as an artifactual reversal of display of the higher velocity signals from an area of flow (Fig. 15). These Doppler shift frequencies exceed the Nyquist limit, which equals one half the pulse repetition frequency (PRF) in a pulsed-Doppler instrument. The illusion of reversal of flow results when not enough samples can be obtained in a given time period to represent accurately the physiologic events being observed. An often-cited analogy is the apparent reversal of motion of the wagon wheel spokes in a Western movie; this illusion occurs because the motion picture frame rate is too low to capture the position of the wheel before it completes one or more full revolutions. In pulsed Doppler systems aliasing may occur because the targeted vessel is located too deep to be adequately interrogated at a suitable PRF or because the depth or PRF scale settings are set deeper than necessary for evaluation of a more superficial vessel. When aliasing is present, accurate velocity measurements are difficult to obtain.

Aliasing also occurs in CCDS. When improper scale or baseline settings are used, the high velocity flow may "wrap around" into the other color scale. This

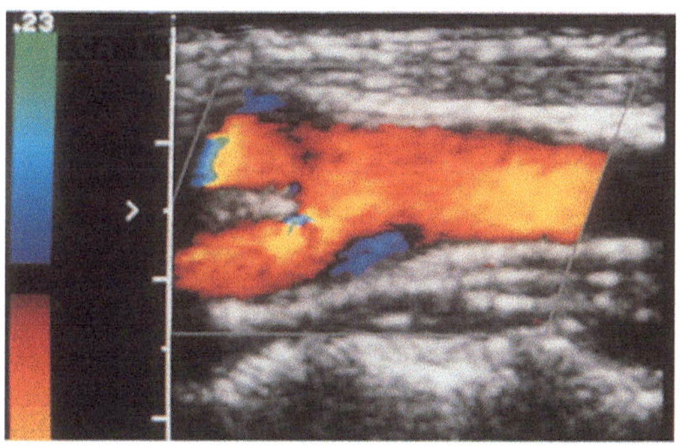
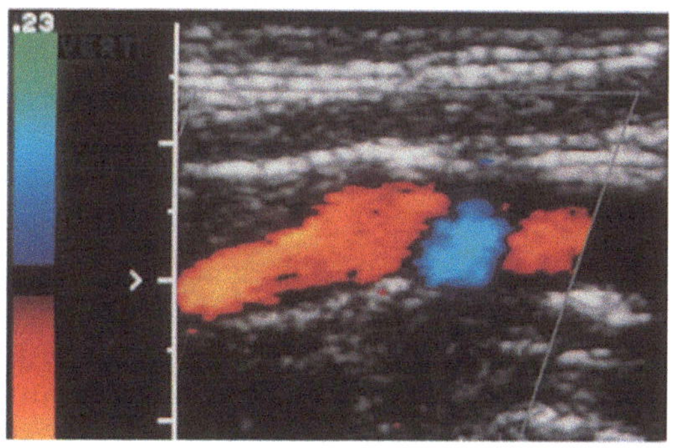

Figs. 13 (left), 14 (right). The great variability in magnitude of flow reversal zones is shown in these two longitudinal CCDS images of the carotid bifurcation area

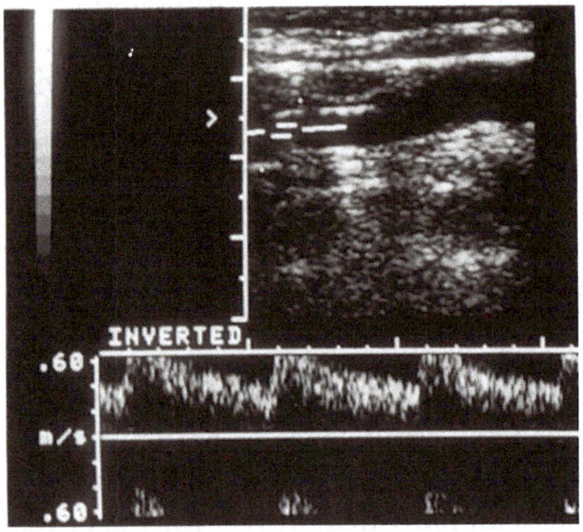

Fig. 15. Aliasing in a duplex spectral tracing: the velocity scale is inadequate to accommodate the high frequency shifts present in the returning Doppler signal; as a result systolic peaks are "wrapped around" on the display

results in a direct change from a red to a blue color. In contrast, true flow reversal also appears as a blue island within the red color-encoded vessel, but it can be differentiated from aliasing by a surrounding black border that represents the "no flow" zone between forward and reversed flow components (Fig. 16). Moreover color saturation is much deeper in true flow reversal because of slow flow within this flow separation area. In a study of Middleton et al., flow reversal could be demonstrated in 99 of 100 carotid arteries in healthy subjects. Therefore it has been proposed that flow reversal at the carotid bifurcation is an expected finding in normal subjects, whereas loss of flow reversal suggests the presence of atheromatous lesions altering the normal carotid bulb configuration. In our own study, however, we could not detect flow reversal in four of 156 patients even though no atheromatous lesions could be found in the bifurcation. In all of these cases no bulb

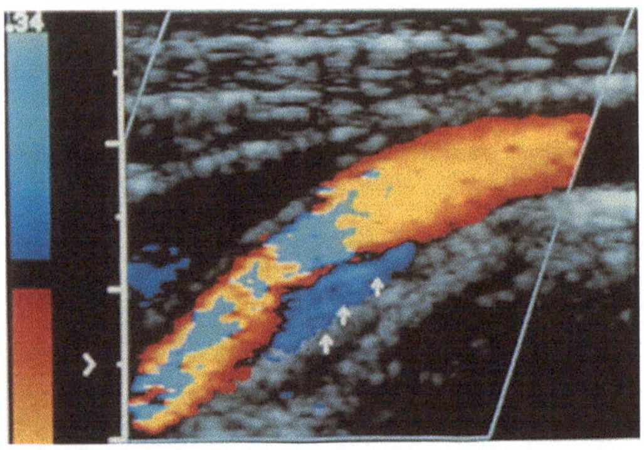

Fig. 16. Aliasing in CCDS: When improper scale or baseline settings are used the high velocity flow may "wrap around" into the other color scale. In this case, it changes directly from a light yellow color to a light blue color. In contrast, true flow reversal (arrows) in this example also appears blue, but it can be differentiated from aliasing by a surrounding black border that represents the "no flow zone" between forward and reversed flow

formation could be demonstrated either in the bifurcation or in the proximal internal carotid artery (Fig. 17). This corresponds well with postmortem studies in which no carotid bulb was found in a small percentage of normal carotid arteries. Thus, we believe that the presence of a carotid bulb is the basis for flow reversal development. On the other hand, flow reversal was demonstrable in several pathological conditions involving the carotid bifurcation. These included patients with several areas of plaque formation within the carotid bifurcation with flow reversal in between the plaques adjacent to the plaque-free vessel wall segment (Fig. 18). A higher probability of progression in atherosclerosis may be assumed in these cases because of associated slow flow velocities in the regions of flow reversal.

The diagnosis of ICA occlusion is easily established with CCDS because of absence of color coding of the occluded segment. Flow reversal is often detectable proximal to the occluded vessel due to the pressure of the blood stream against the occlusion (Fig. 19). From a clinical point of view this observation may be important, since patients with ICA occlusion and a large flow reversal proximal to the occlusion (stump syndrome) are significantly more likely to develop symptoms of cerebral ischemia during follow up. This supports the concept of embolization from

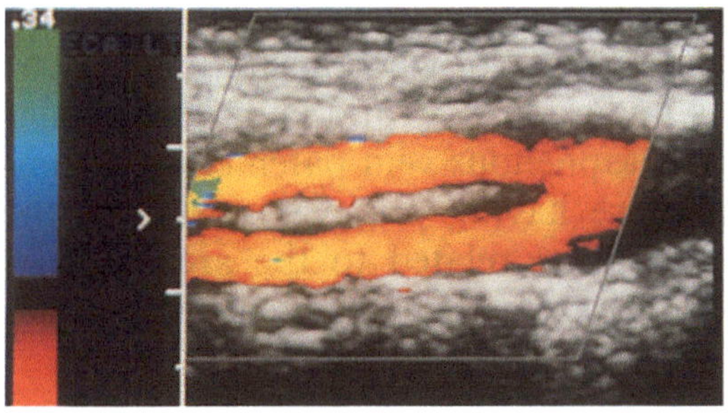

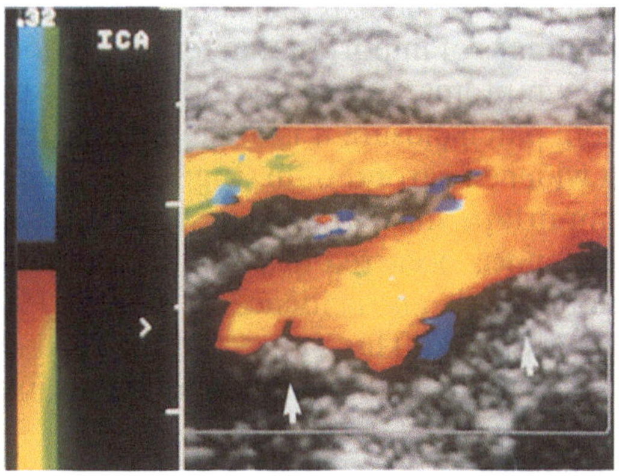

Fig. 17. (left) Longitudinal sonogram of carotid bifurcation and proximal portions of ICA and ECA shows normal morphologic and hemodynamic appearance. However, no bulb formation is identified in the CCA or ICA

Fig. 18. (right) Longitudinal view of carotid bifurcation illustrating a flow reversal zone in a plaque-free segment of the posterior vessel wall surrounded by atheromatous calcified plaques (arrows)

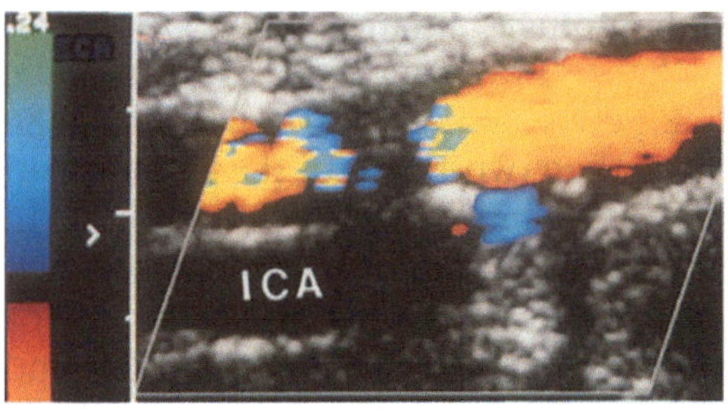

Fig. 19. No color flow within the ICA lumen can be demonstrated in this longitudinal sonogram, indicating occlusion of the vessel. Flow reversal is shown proximal to the occlusion. A medium-grade stenosis of the ECA is also displayed

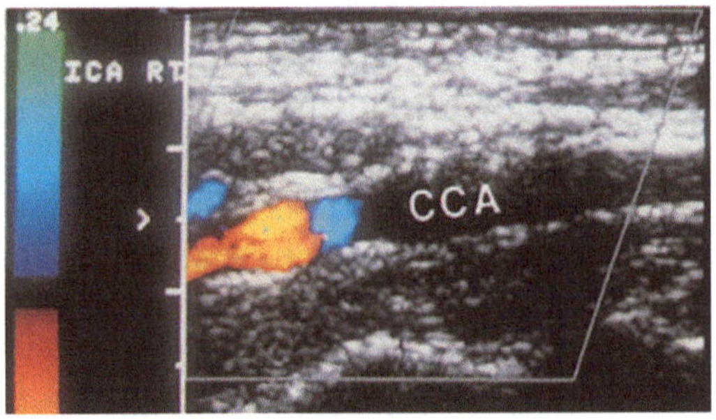

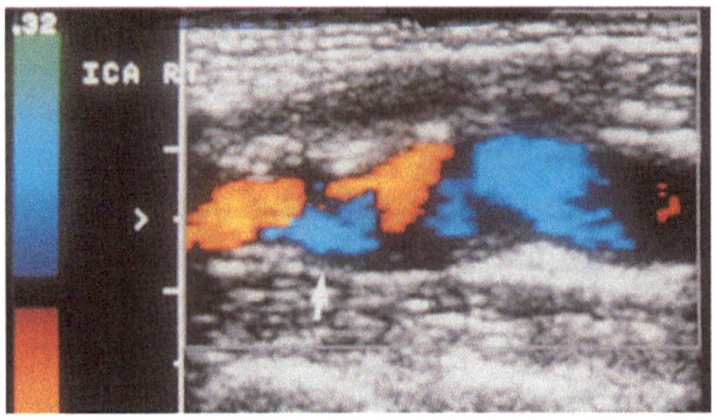

Fig. 20. (left) Longitudinal view of CCA and carotid bifurcation demonstrates absence of color flow and material of low echogenicity filling the lumen of the CCA in a case of CCA occlusion. Distal to the occluded CCA a flow reversal zone is shown, indicating a patent carotid bifurcation

Fig. 21. (right) Status post ICA thrombendarterectomy: this longitudinal view documents widening of the vessel lumen (enlarged bulb-like formation) after saphenous vein patch closure; large areas of flow reversal are noted (arrow)

the carotid bifurcation as a cause of episodic cerebral ischemia following ICA occlusion.

With occlusion of the CCA, flow reversal is observed in the carotid bifurcation when both the external and internal carotid branches are patent (Fig. 20). This finding is of importance in terms of choosing between possible treatment modalities in symptomatic patients. Following carotid endarterectomy utilizing a saphenous vein patch closure it is often possible to demonstrate large areas of flow reversal in a widened carotid bulb (Fig. 21). From a clinical point of view this finding may be important since in a large series of patients undergoing carotid endarterectomies restenosis occurred in 13% of patients having saphenous vein patch closure compared with an incidence of only 1.7% in those having primary closure of the arteriotomy. This suggests that thrombus build-up related to the area of flow reversal at the patch site may be an important risk factor for restenosis.

Plaque morphology

The primary objective of carotid endarterectomy is the prevention of strokes. In principle, flow-reducing carotid stenoses with ipsilateral symptoms are accepted criteria for selection of patients for carotid endarterectomy. The optimal management of carotid lesions *not* associated with symptoms is a major source of controversy. Central to this controversy is that the natural course of asymptomatic carotid disease is not well defined. Javid et al. performed serial arteriograms in 86 patients with documented carotid disease. More than two-thirds of the patients had progression of the disease, with one-third increasing more than 25% each year. In a study by Sterpetti et al. the overall incidence of new neurologic events associated with diameter reduction greater than 50% was 19%, with an incidence of 10% for TIA and 9% for stroke. Moore et al. retrospectively studied 303 patients and found a significant correlation between incidence of stroke and severity of stenosis. Of 109 patients, 21 (19%) with diameter stenosis greater than 50% suffered strokes during a follow-up period of 5 years. Hertzer et al. reviewed the course of 195 unoperated patients who had carotid disease exceeding 50% reduction in lumen diameter and who had no symptoms. The 5-year incidence of focal neurologic deficits was 22%. They found that the incidence of stroke was higher among those who had at least 70% unilateral stenosis. The presence of significant stenosis bilaterally, arterial hypertension, evidence of coronary artery disease and history of smoking are regarded as significant risk factors. The prevalence and severity of carotid disease is related to age, which is the most important risk factor for stroke. Yet the prevalence of 50% or greater diameter stenosis, even in the oldest population groups studied, has proved low. Of 722 individuals examined in the Framingham study, with a mean age of 75 years, only 9% had lumen diameter narrowing of 50% or greater. Thus, the changes responsible for TIA's and strokes must be sought on the basis of more subtle plaque analysis (as well as identification of other potential sources of emboli related to cardiac pathology, etc.).

The use of high-resolution B-mode real-time sonography offers a unique opportunity to define carotid plaque in terms of echogenicity, giving clues to the structure of the plaque and, eventually, determining differences among types of plaques. In a multivariate analysis only the severity of stenosis and the presence of heterogeneous plaques were independent risk factors. Reilly et al., Bluth et al. and O'Donnell et al. have been able to identify lesions with intraplaque hemorrhage noninvasively with over 95% sensitivity and 87% specificity by noting heterogeneous soft echodensities in the sonographic image of the plaques. In a study by Weinberger et al. 97% of hemorrhagic plaques were heterogeneous on ultrasonography and 77% of heterogeneous plaques contained intraplaque hemorrhage on pathology, while 23% had degenerative changes without recent hemorrhage. Intraluminal thrombus overlying plaque was only seen in association with intraplaque hemorrhages. It is possible that intraluminal thrombus over carotid plaques is a source of emboli to the cerebral circulation. The detection of intraplaque hemorrhage by ultrasound may be of clinical importance since Imparato et al. and Lusby et al. have found an increased frequency of transient and permanent cerebral symptoms ipsilateral to carotid plaques with intramural hemorrhage. Lusby et al. found a 92.5% frequency of intraplaque hemorrhage in symptomatic lesions, compared to a 27% frequency in asymptomatic lesions. Imparato et al. found that 82% of lesions with intraplaque hemorrhage were associated with ipsilateral symptoms, while 62% of fibrous plaques were associated with ipsilateral symptoms, a significant difference. Overall plaque echogenicity has been reported to be predictive of ischemic neurologic symptoms in carotid arteries with less than 75% stenosis, with hypoechoic plaques having greater predictive value for the development of transient ischemic attack or stroke. In addition to possible sonographic demonstration of intraplaque hemorrhage, the inverse relationship between plaque lipid content and echogenicity is promising in light of a report of significantly greater total lipid and cholesterol content in symptomatic endarterectomy specimens vs. asymptomatic specimens. Furthermore, an association has been made between cervical carotid plaque ulceration and cerebral emboli. However, angiographic sensitivity for ulceration has been disappointing and conclusive studies establishing the accuracy of ultrasound for detection of ulceration have not yet been published.

Bo, McKinney, et al. observed extensive proliferation of the vasa vasorum in a study of atherosclerotic carotid bifurcations from 8 of 12 non-embalmed cadavers (ages 40–96 at time of death). The small vessels were found to arise primarily from external carotid artery branches (superior thyroid and ascending pharyngeal). This

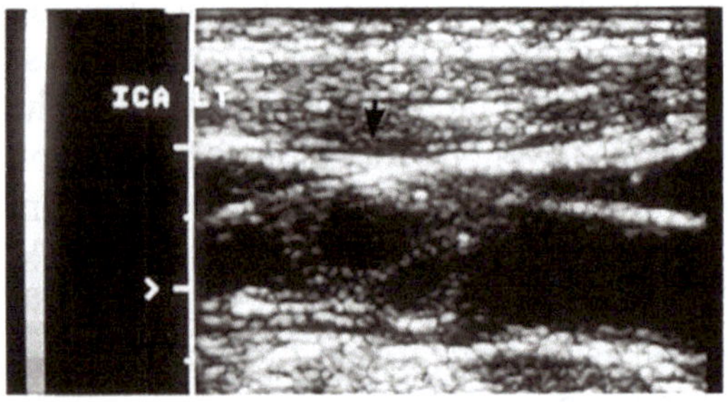

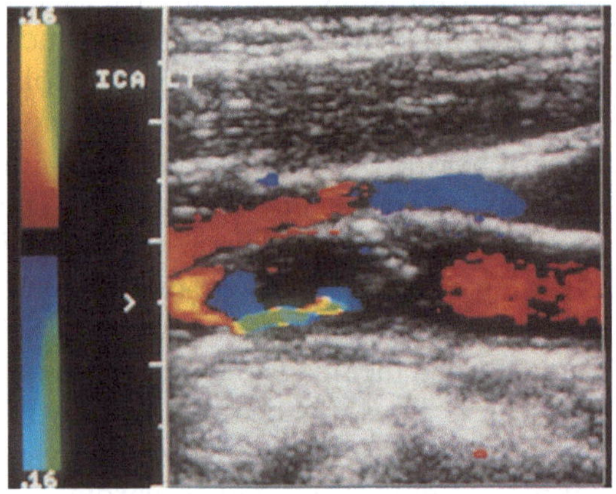

Fig. 22. (left) B-mode imaging of carotid bifurcation demonstrates heterogeneous material filling the lumen and suggesting probable vessel occlusion; several echolucent areas suggestive of intraplaque hemorrhage are present (arrow)

Fig. 23. (right) CCDS in the same plane as Fig. 22 reveals a filiform residual lumen, demonstrating that the occlusion is actually subtotal

study suggests that angiogenic factors may be involved in plaque development; macrophages and platelets are known to play a role in plaque generation and are also known to have angiogenic properties. In the 4 cadavers without significant atherosclerotic changes at the bifurcation no vessel proliferation was shown. The authors suggest that compromised flow in external carotid branch vessels may be a factor in ischemic and hemorrhagic changes within areas of plaque in view of the origin of the vasa vasorum from the external system.

By means of CCDS an excellent delineation of vessel wall irregularities is possible, even in cases of low-echodensity plaques or thrombus formation which might go undetected on conventional B-mode images. The color-coded Doppler signal at the lesion site improves the evaluation of the extent of carotid plaques by the simultaneous two-dimensional display of tissue characteristics (structure) and the flow velocity profile (Figs. 22, 23). One reason for this is that atherosclerotic

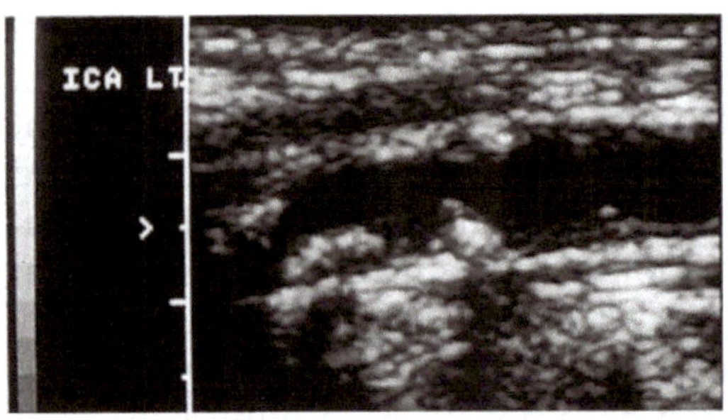

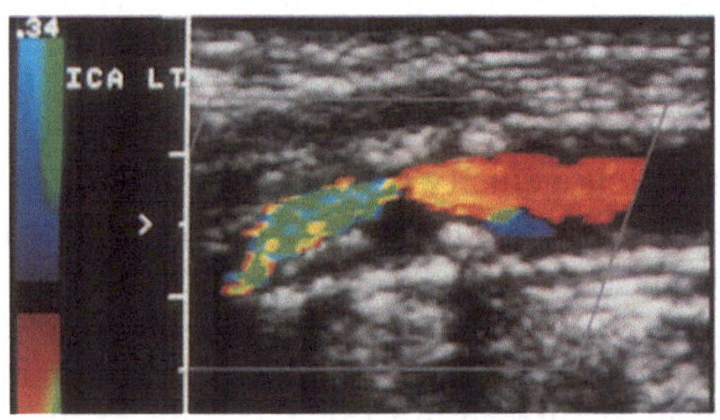

Figs. 24 (left), 25 (right). B-mode imaging shows calcified plaques on the posterior wall of the ICA with only mild stenosis suggested. CCDS reveals only a narrow band of color in the patent portion of the vessel lumen, documenting the presence of a large anechoic plaque, not visible on B-mode, between calcified plaques. This high-grade stenosis could easily have been missed without the additional information provided by color imaging

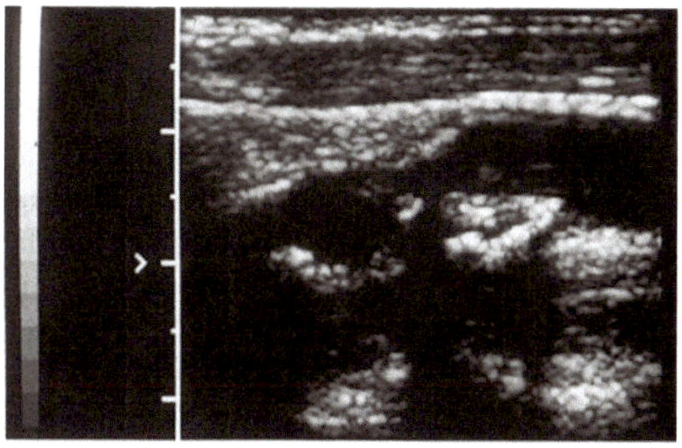

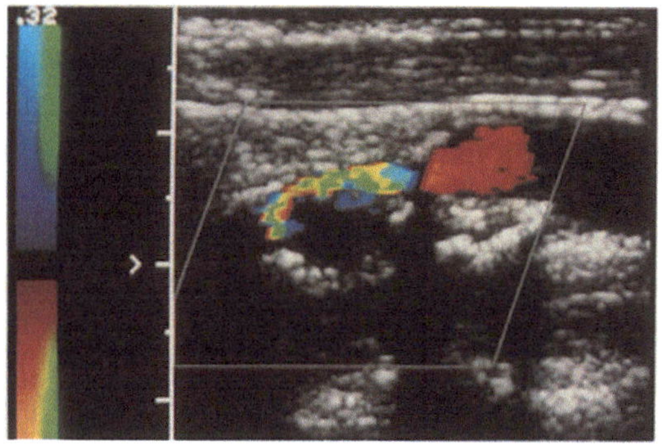

Figs. 26 (left), 27 (right). B-mode imaging shows small calcified plaques on the posterior ICA wall. No significant stenosis was suspected. Distal to the visible plaques color flow reveals a large anechoic plaque causing marked stenosis with flow velocity increase and post-stenotic turbulence

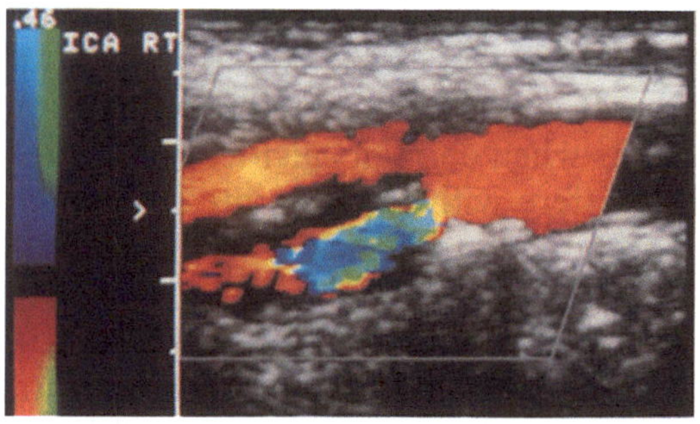

Fig. 28. Longitudinal sonogram of carotid bifurcation demonstrates a small, homogeneous, thorn-like plaque on the posterior wall with marked flow disturbance downstream from the plaque

plaques are more conspicuous with CCDS when outlined against the color flow lumen (Figs. 24, 25). Another more important reason is the ability to assess directly anechoic plaque components such as necrotic and thrombotic material, which now can be identified adjacent to the vessel wall and the atherosclerotic plaque due to absence of the color-flow signal despite the lack of gray-scale signals (Figs. 26, 27). Third, CCDS reveals circumscribed, peri-atheromatous flow disturbances in a majority of small plaques (of interest due to the theoretically higher risk of emboli from plaques with irregular surface characteristics) (Fig. 28). Detection of these local alterations in flow patterns and differentiating the findings from complex blood flow variants in the normal carotid bifurcation is difficult using only standard duplex analysis, a major drawback to generalized application of this analysis technique. Despite the advantage of standard non-invasive tests for the evaluation of carotid disease, this lack of simultaneous display of the morphologic-hemodynamic interaction of carotid lesions has until now been a major handicap in carrying out prospective follow-up investigations. With conventional sonography, the degree of stenosis may be underestimated when the atherosclerotic plaque is partly anechoic.

The ability of CCDS to facilitate differentiation of smooth and irregular surface structures and identification of ulcerative niches is of great clinical importance, since recent evidence suggests that most cerebrovascular events are likely to be of embolic origin and the vascular source of many previously undetectable embolic events now may be identifiable. Prospective evaluation of repair mechanisms as well as progression of small and intermediate-sized plaques is also facilitated; this may influence risk factor adjustment and medical treatment in individual patients.

In summary, high-resolution sonography assisted by color-flow imaging promises a higher accuracy in plaque structure analysis, particularly if the plaque contains one or more large focal sonolucent areas; detection of plaque ulceration should also be facilitated.

Stenosis

Atherosclerotic lesions are most commonly found in the carotid bifurcation and proximal ICA; lesions limited to the ECA are found in only 13% of cases, and in the CCA in 1–2%. Atherosclerosis affecting the posterior (dorsal) aspect of the ICA wall is found in 55% and at the bifurcation in 25%. The lateral wall segment of the ICA is involved in 35% and the bifurcation in 20%. Anterior (ventral) location of plaques is found in 14% in the ICA and 13% at the bifurcation. Anterior location of plaque may pose problems when enough calcification is present to cause posterior shadowing; this can interfere with the accurate assignment of color flow map data in the affected region and lead to difficulty in the accurate grading of stenosis (Figs. 29, 30).

Numerous studies have evaluated the ability of sonography to determine with accuracy the degree of carotid stenosis. Methods include the use of real-time sonography to measure the percentage of diameter reduction and the use of duplex Doppler for measurement of flow velocities and velocity ratios as well as assessment of the degree of spectral broadening. B-mode imaging has been used mainly for precise placement of the sample volume for Doppler waveform acquisition to allow grading of stenosis related to flow velocity. The Doppler velocity criteria have been shown to be less accurate when reduction in ICA diameter is under 50%. Furthermore, assessment of spectral broadening in the evaluation of low-grade lesions is extremely dependent on the use of appropriate receiver gain settings.

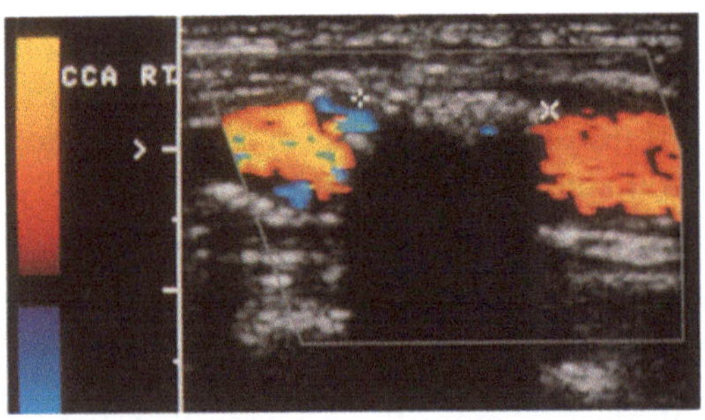

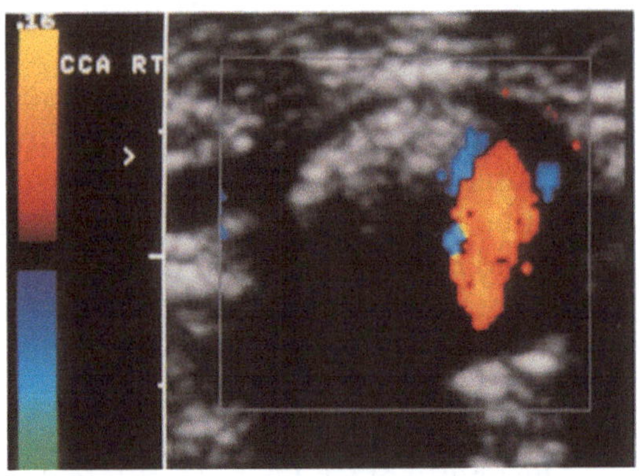

Figs. 29 (left), 30 (right). Longitudinal and transverse sonograms of proximal ICA show an extensive, calcified plaque formation on the anterior wall of the vessel with broad distal shadowing. Because of this no Doppler signal and no useful color flow information can be obtained

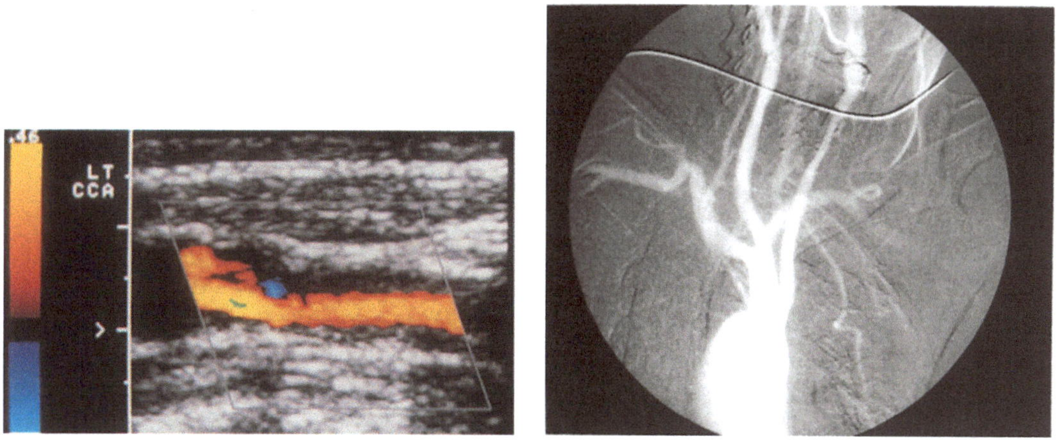

a *b*

Fig. 31. ***a*** CCDS shows a long segment of lumen narrowing in the CCA due to diffuse thickening of the vascular wall without significant increase in flow velocity or presence of turbulence. ***b*** Angiography of same patient

Duplex sonography of the carotids is a technically demanding and time-consuming procedure. Real-time B-scanning can show a relatively large segment of the vessel wall and lumen, but Doppler assessment of flow disturbances and increased flow velocity can be obtained only from one small area at a time. Conventional sonography cannot consistently define the residual lumen; because of this, grading of stenoses often relies on Doppler criteria alone. Doppler criteria (flow velocity measurements) on the other hand are limited in high-flow or slow-flow states such as hypertension, congestive heart failure, tortuosity, and carotid dissection. Doppler criteria can be misleading in the presence of a contralateral high-grade stenosis or occlusion; a gradually tapering stenosis may also be underestimated because of minimal turbulence and a persistently normal flow velocity. This is often observed in the CCA with a semicircular or concentric stenosis, where duplex Doppler or CCDS may show a normal flow pattern without increase in flow velocity and turbulence even when CCA stenosis of up to 60% by area is present (Fig. 31). When hemodynamically insignificant lesions are located in the carotid bulb, arterial flow velocities are frequently normal, presumably because the carotid bulb can accommodate a large plaque while maintaining a flow lumen comparable to that of the CCA proximally and the ICA distally. In such cases no flow velocity changes (other than a potential loss of the pattern of flow reversal normally associated with the bulb area) may be present, and angiography may give no indication of plaque formation. In such cases B-mode imaging may delineate the true dimensions of the bulb and its associated plaque while CCDS documents the flow lumen and the absence of flow closer to the true vessel wall.

Despite these limitations continuous-wave Doppler and single-gate pulsed-wave Doppler sonography combined in duplex systems are reported to be accurate relative to angiography for the detection of obstruction producing a narrowing of the lumen greater then 50%. Exact classification of subgroups within this "greater than 50%" population has proved relatively less accurate in most studies: Hennerici et al. misclassified 37% of obstructive lesions with lumen narrowings of greater than 50% when using a multigate pulsed-wave Doppler system. Glover et al.

reported agreement of duplex and angiographic estimates in 54% of cases with stenosis in the 30–70% range; Roederer et al. reported a concordance of 86% for 50–79% stenosis, but only 71% for 80–99% stenoses. Fell et al. found a correct estimation in only 72% of 50–99% stenoses and Zwiebel et al. over- or undergraded 31% of carotid stenoses. Jacobs et al. found the overall accuracy of duplex scanning improved during the course of their study; after 6 months 89% of 51–90% stenoses were classified correctly.

The sensitivity of color Doppler for the detection of carotid disease is reported to be 100% when compared with angiography. The accuracy of color Doppler in classifying minimal (40–60%), moderate (61–80%) and severe (81–99%) stenosis ranged from 91.3% to 97.8% compared to angiography; this is slightly better than the comparable accuracy rates of 91.7% to 95.8% reported for conventional Doppler sonography. Color flow can help direct attention to areas of stenosis within a vessel for a more detailed duplex examination. Precise placement of the Doppler sample volume is facilitated by availability of the simultaneous color image of the vessel lumen. Angle correction has to be performed relative to the course of the residual lumen rather than the vessel wall. For quantitative Doppler measurements we apply the multicenter recommendation for standardized imaging and Doppler criteria by Bluth et al. (see Table p. 49). Peak systolic velocity (PSV) and peak end-diastolic velocity (PEDV) are measured at the point of maximum stenosis (Figs. 32, 33). The peak systolic velocity ratio (SVR) and peak diastolic velocity ratio (DVR) are the peak systolic (diastolic) velocity at the point of maximum stenosis in the ICA divided by the peak systolic (diastolic) velocity in the unobstructed CCA one centimeter or more below the bifurcation. These velocity ratios provide information about the degree of stenosis which is less dependent on absolute individual flow velocities. Turbulence results in an increased range (distribution) of flow velocities which is referred to as "spectral broadening". Spectral broadening should be determined distal to the stenosis and is usually measured at peak systole (Fig. 34). Spectral broadening can be quantified by measuring

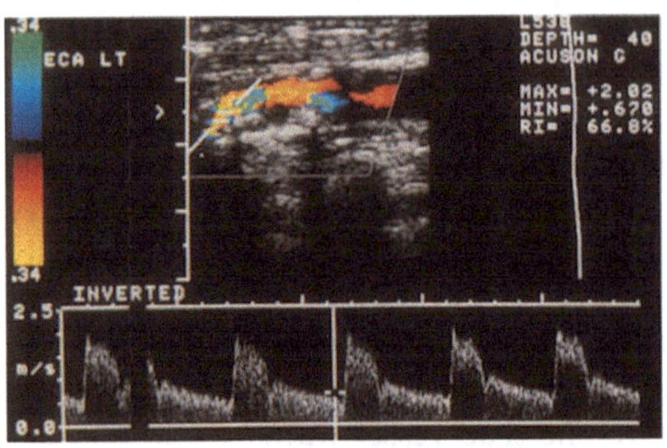

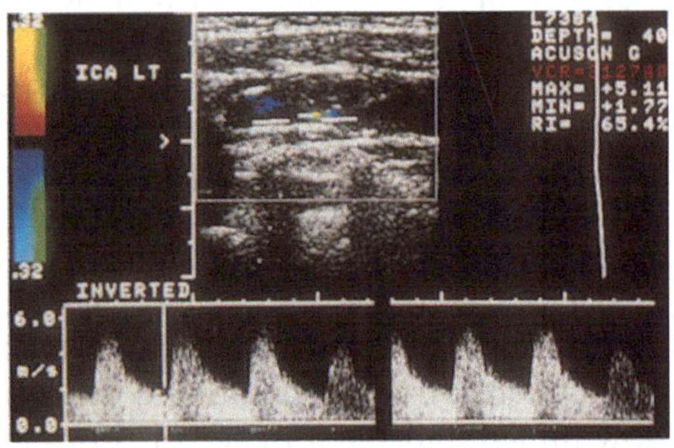

Fig. 32 (left). Longitudinal sonogram of carotid bifurcation and ICA shows calcified plaques in carotid bulb and origin of ICA. Spectral tracing shows angle-corrected peak systolic and end-diastolic velocities of 2.02 and 0.67 m/sec. This corresponds to a grade 3 (60–79%) stenosis (see Table p. 49)

Fig. 33 (right). This longitudinal sonogram shows high-grade stenosis involving the proximal ICA with heterogeneous plaques and a residual color-coded lumen adjacent to the posterior wall. Spectral tracing displays peak systolic and end-diastolic flow velocities of 5.1 and 1.8 m/sec with marked spectral broadening consistent with a grade 4 stenosis (80–99%)

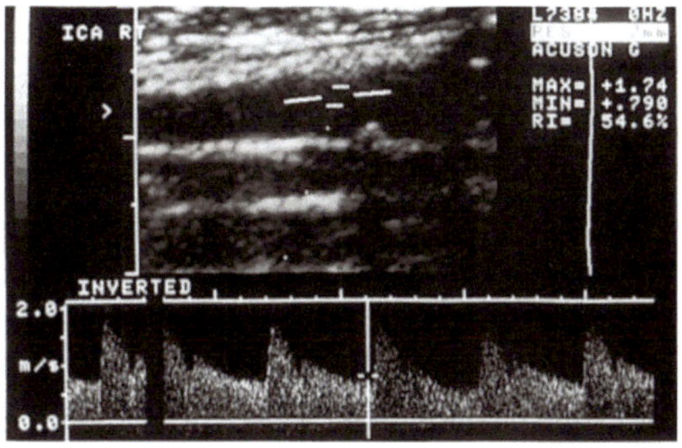

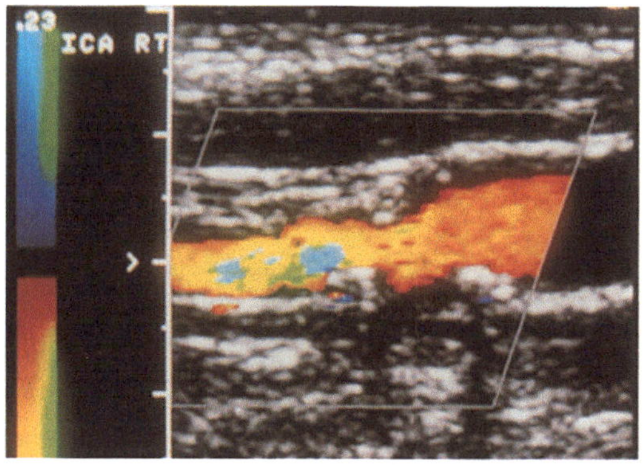

Fig. 34. (left) Duplex Doppler sonography spectral tracing obtained at the level of the carotid bifurcation and proximal ICA shows broad bandwidth with a partially "filled in" systolic envelope (spectral broadening) representing turbulent flow

Fig. 35. (right) CCDS showing 40% area stenosis of the ICA with decreased color saturation indicating increased flow velocity. This stenosis is due to a long-segment plaque on the posterior wall

the range of velocities at the 50% amplitude level of the Doppler power spectrum (histogram).

Qualitative classification of ICA stenosis is also possible based on CCDS findings. In low-grade stenosis (40–60% by area) typical findings include a long segment of increased flow velocity (decreased color saturation during systole), minimal post-stenotic turbulence, and relatively little plaque extent on B-mode (Fig. 35). Medium-grade stenosis (61–80% by area) is characterized by increased systolic and diastolic flow velocity (decreased color saturation during systole and diastole), turbulent and reversed post-stenotic flow, and moderate lumen narrowing on the B-mode image (Fig. 36). High-grade (81–99% by area) stenosis results in a short segment of marked reduction of color saturation ("color fading"), severe post-stenotic flow reversal and turbulence, severe lumen narrowing on B-mode, and reduced pre-stenotic flow velocity in the CCA (Fig. 37).

The fact that even in the transverse plane an adequate color-flow image of the vessels can be obtained allows measuring percentage of stenosis with CCDS. For this purpose, we directly compared residual lumen with vessel area at the same level in the internal carotid artery. This measurement, the percent area stenosis, is defined as (1 minus the residual lumen area/vessel lumen area) × 100 where vessel lumen area is determined by circumferential measurement of the vessel wall and residual lumen area is determined by corresponding measurement at the color flow boundary of the residual lumen (Figs. 38, 39). The direct residual area (percent stenosis) measurement corresponds to what has traditionally been used in angiographic determination of ICA stenosis and has the additional advantage of a transverse plane, which better represents the configuration of the stenosing plaque. This is of great importance in accurate assessment of eccentric stenosis, where a more correct anatomic estimate of the percentage of stenosis is possible than with the measurement technique used in the DSA examinations (drawing 2). The fact that there is a cephaled oblique component of angulation relative to the true cross section of the vessel on simultaneous color/B-mode display does not adversely influence the accuracy of percent stenosis estimate since both areas are equally affected.

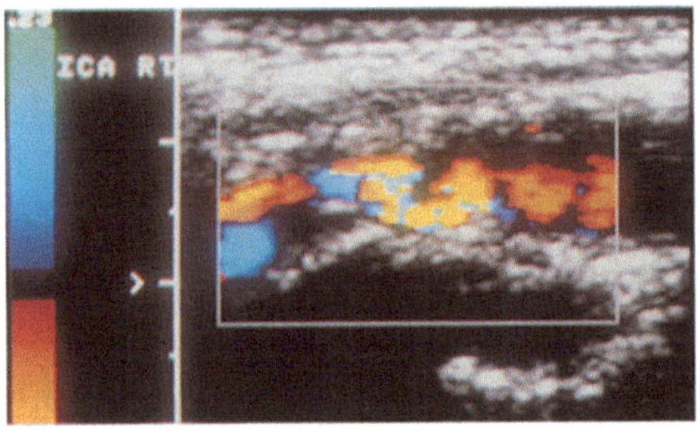

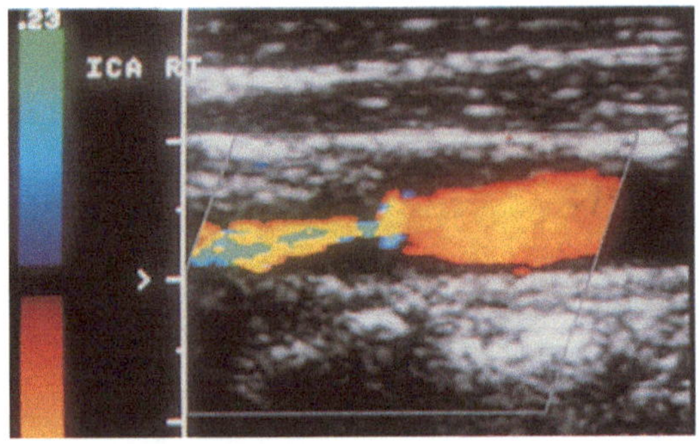

Fig. 36. (left) CCDS shows a heterogeneous plaque formation on the anterior wall of ICA producing a 60% stenosis with marked decrease in color saturation indicating increased flow velocity; moderate post-stenotic mixed color pattern indicates the presence of velocity variance compatible with turbulent flow

Fig. 37. (right) CCDS of a high-grade stenosis of ICA (85% area stenosis) with short segment of maximum reduction in color saturation followed by marked post-stenotic turbulence and flow reversal

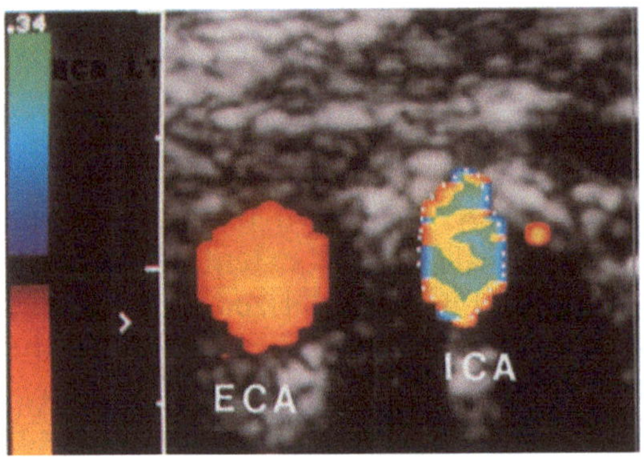

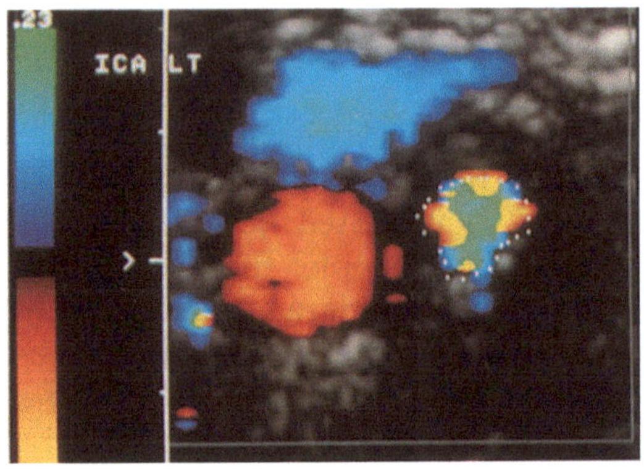

Fig. 38. (left) Transverse CCDS of ICA demonstrates an area stenosis of 65% with eccentric residual lumen, decreased color saturation, and mixed color pattern representing areas of high flow velocity and turbulence; contrast these findings with the normal appearance of the ECA in the same view

Fig. 39. (right) Another example of area stenosis measurement (75%) of an irregular area of ICA narrowing

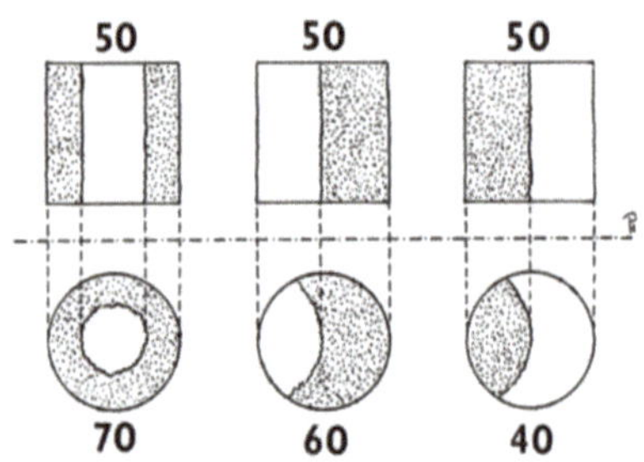

drawing 2

In a study of Erickson et al. the percentage of diameter stenosis of the ICA was estimated directly from color Doppler images obtained in both longitudinal and transverse planes and compared with the results of digital substraction angiography. Percent diameter stenosis could not be determined in 12% of color Doppler flow imaging studies due to calcified plaques. Percent diameter stenosis determined by CCDS was greater than by angiography in 25% of cases and less in 4%. When the percentages of diameter reduction estimated with velocity criteria from the ICA were compared with direct measurements from the CCDS images, findings were found to be similiar to those previously described with conventional duplex Doppler vs. selective angiography.

Pathologic conditions in the CCA are easily assessed with CCDS. In patients with abnormal enlargement of the CCA lumen, hemodynamic changes due to altered vessel geometry include reduced blood flow and marked flow reversal near the vascular wall. The narrowing of a long segment of the CCA lumen up to the bifurcation is usually caused by a concentric, diffuse thickening of the vessel wall which does not lead to significant hemodynamic alterations (Fig. 40).

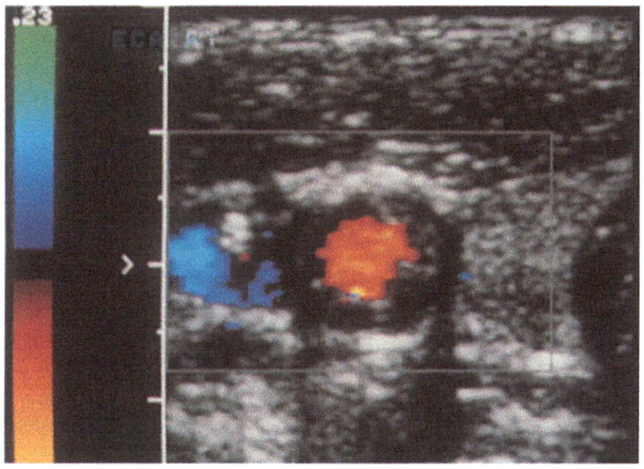

Fig. 40. Transverse sonogram of CCA shows a concentric stenosis with atheromatous lesions of low echodensity and irregular surface characteristics. The color-coded residual lumen shows no evidence of increased flow velocity or turbulence

High-grade stenosis and subtotal occlusion

CCDS is useful in differentiating high-grade stenoses from occlusions. With high-grade stenosis a "string" of color flow corresponding to a very narrow column of flowing blood in the stenotic segment may be seen; flow velocity may be increased or even decreased along this small channel (Fig. 41). Such a filiform stenosis can easily be missed with duplex scanning if the sample volume is not placed in precisely the correct position. This can result in the false impression of a complete occlusion when a surgically correctable high-grade stenosis is actually present. Scanning with color flow in a transverse plane can show even a tiny lumen with relatively slow flow (Fig. 42). When the artery gradually becomes stenosed, flow (cross-sectional area × velocity) is reduced when the diameter is decreased by 50–70%; flow *velocity,* however, continues to increase until the diameter is reduced by about 90% (drawing 3). With further stenosis, flow velocity begins to decrease as the jet is almost turned off. While the frequency shift gradually returns to normal or even lower than normal, progressive distortion of the duplex Doppler spectral waveform allows differentiation from a normal vessel. The importance of CCDS is that it allows a further increase in the sensitivity of detection of extremely slow flow. Even pseudo-occlusion of the ICA (a condition that is characterized by flow velocities

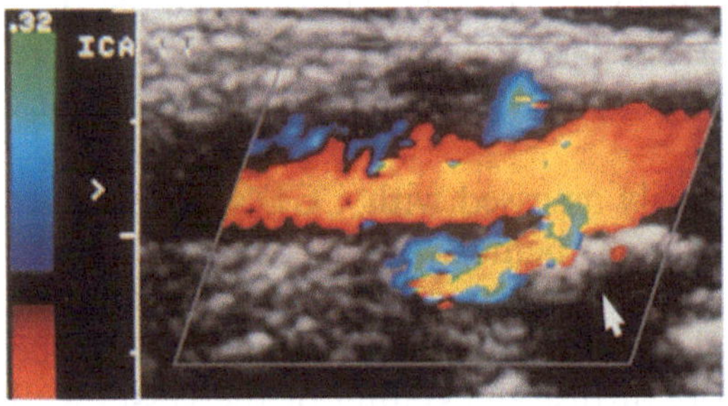

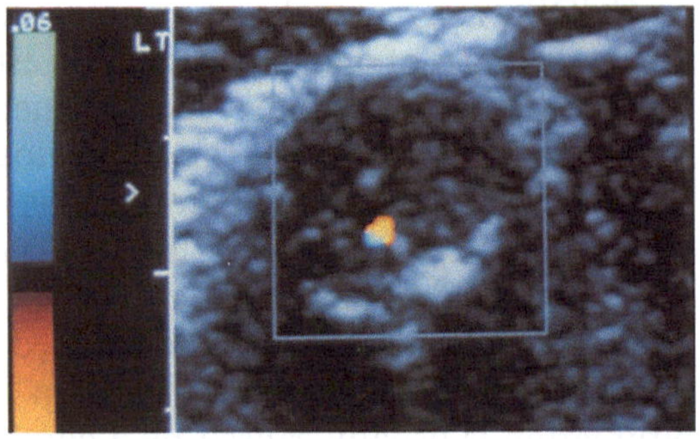

Fig. 41. (left) CCDS of carotid bifurcation shows high-grade stenosis of the ICA with resultant flow jet; the plaque is heavily calcified (arrow)

Fig. 42. (right) On this magnified transverse ICA image a very small color-coded lumen, representing minimal residual flow, can be seen within the vessel which is filled with low-echodensity material; without color flow imaging vessel occlusion was suggested

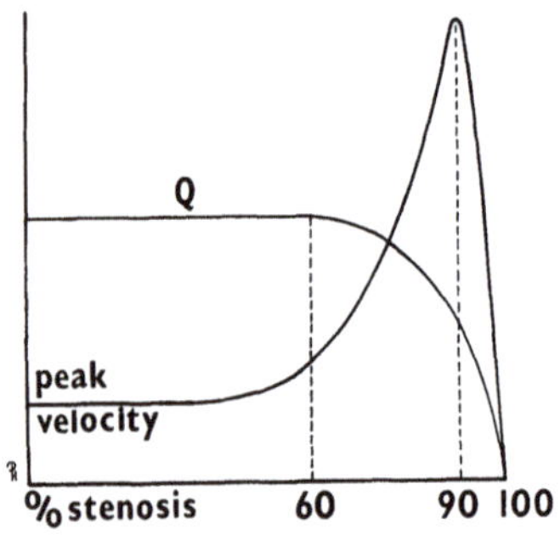

drawing 3

equal to zero distal to a very tight stenosis or segmental occlusion with retrograde filling from the siphon) is detectable by CCDS. Until recently the detection of this vascular condition was restricted to the use of special angiographic techniques of transfemoral subtraction angiography with selective carotid (and sometimes vertebral) catheterization and occasionally long serial imaging runs of reduced flow rates and increased injection bolus requirements.

If the ICA is stenosed by more than 90% or occluded, collateral vessels connecting it with the ECA system may develop spontaneously or be created surgically (extracranial-intracranial bypass) (Figs. 68, 69, 70). In either case, because the ECA now represents a low resistance vascular bed with increased flow, its waveform may appear "internalized" (sloping gradually toward the baseline during diastole with an increase in diastolic flow velocity, as generally expected in the internal carotid artery). This may be anticipated based on an "externalized" CCA with a rapid upstroke during systole and a rapid return to baseline during diastole, since it now supplies mainly the ECA and its branches (Fig. 43). CCDS shows increased pulsatility of the CCA (no color-coding during diastole) and decreased pulsatility in the ECA (continuous display of color throughout the cardiac cycle).

Signs of ICA occlusion include absence of color coding of the lumen even with high sensitivity "slow-flow" velocity settings (Figs. 44, 45), a marked decrease in relative diastolic flow in the ipsilateral CCA in comparison to the opposite carotid, and an early diastolic flow reversal at the ICA origin, which is easily discernible with CCDS (Fig. 46).

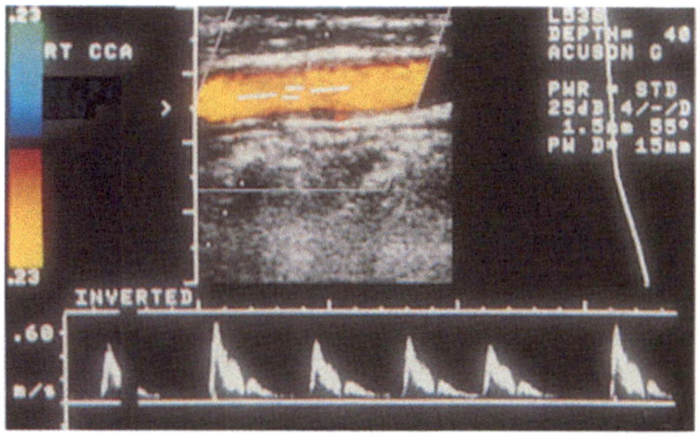

Fig. 43. Spectral tracing from the CCA shows an "externalized" flow pattern with a rapid upstroke during systole and a rapid return to baseline during diastole; this pattern is typically associated with severe stenosis or occlusion of the ipsilateral ICA

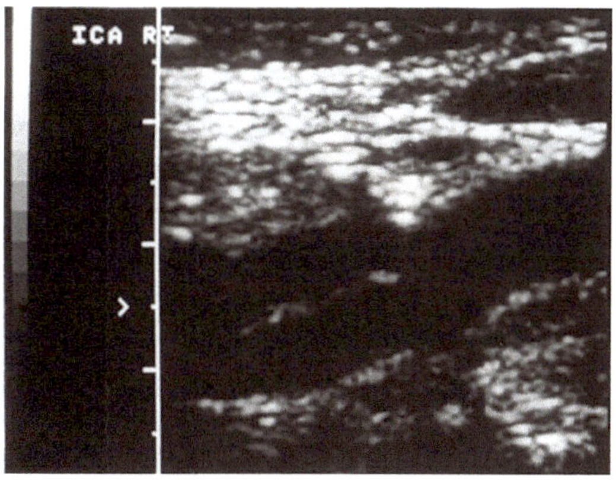

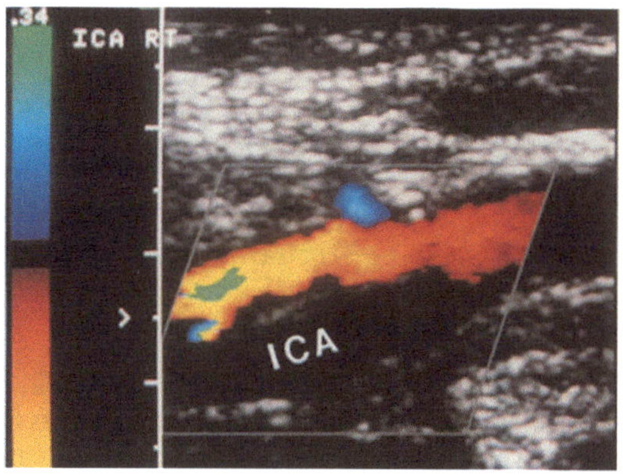

Figs. 44 (left), 45 (right). B-mode image of carotid bifurcation appears normal, but absence of color flow in the ICA correctly identifies occlusion due to anechoic material

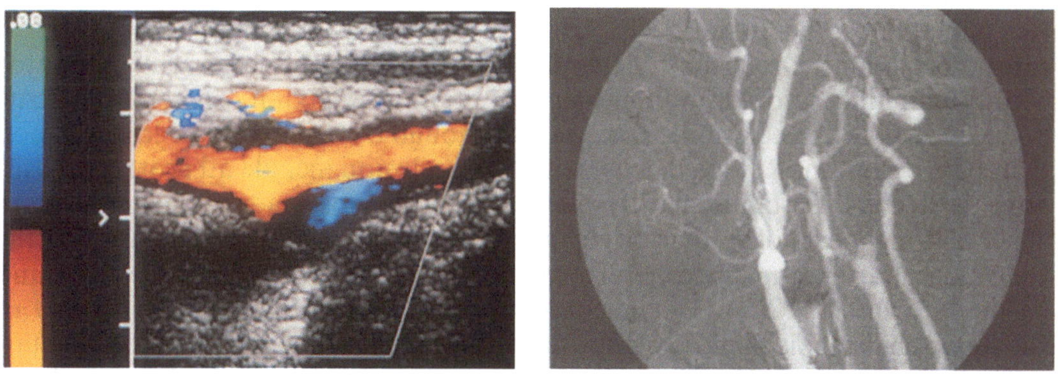

a *b*

Fig. 46. ***a*** CCDS shows total ICA occlusion with flow reversal just proximal to the occluded segment. ***b*** Angiography of same patient

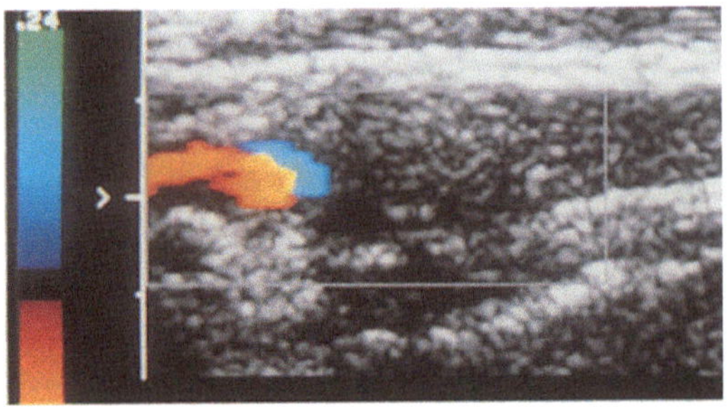

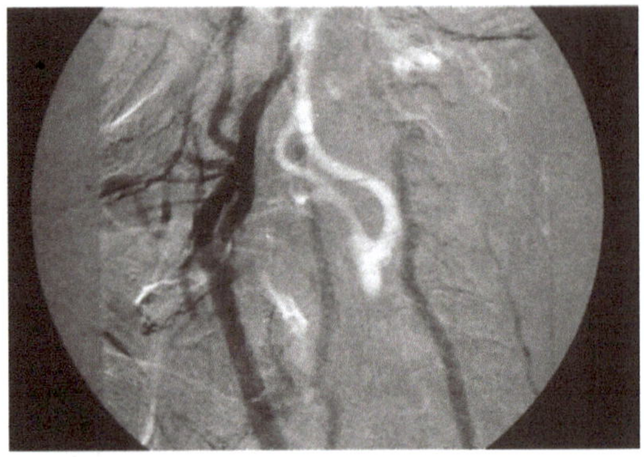

a *b*

Fig. 47. ***a*** CCDS demonstrates a long-segment occlusion of the CCA with echogenic material filling the lumen; color flow signals from the bifurcation indicate patency of carotid branches. ***b*** Angiography of same patient

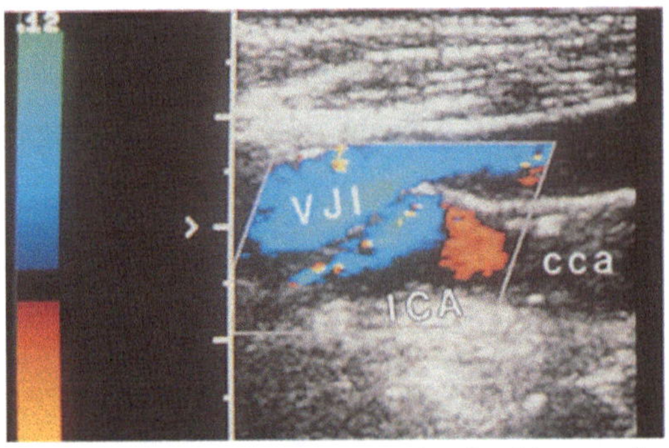

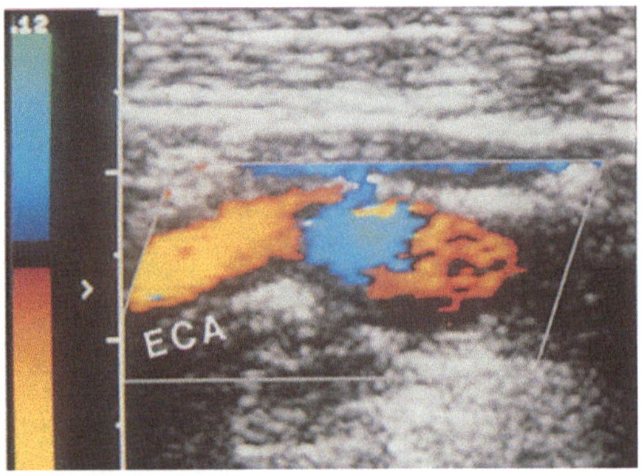

Figs. 48 (left), 49 (right). Longitudinal images in a case of CCA occlusion demonstrate a patent ICA with reversed flow (blue) and ECA with antegrade flow (red)

In cases of total CCA occlusion CCDS is useful in determining whether or not the ipsilateral ICA and ECA are still patent (Figs. 47, 48, 49). The incidence of CCA occlusion in patients suffering cerebral ischemia due to atherosclerotic lesions is estimated to vary from less than 1% to 5%. Dyken et al. reviewed 279 consecutive angiograms and found 5 (1.8%) CCA occlusions and 38 (13.6%) internal carotid occlusions. Occlusions of the ICA and CCA are not necessarily associated with cerebral infarction or even measurable brain dysfunction. Therefore the true prevalence of CCA occlusion is uncertain, although it is known to be less common than ICA occlusion. Reported causes of CCA occlusion include atherothrombosis, arteritis, aortitis, fibromuscular dysplasia, thrombocytosis, aortic arch dissection, aneurysm, embolism of cardiac origin, and craniocervical trauma. Occlusion of the CCA is usually accompanied by propagation of the thrombus into the ECA and particularly into the ICA. Documentation of ECA and ICA patency by way of collateral channels is clinically important since a subclavian-carotid or carotid-carotid bypass in such cases may relieve symptoms of cerebral hemispheric ischemia. In the presence of CCA occlusion, routine angiography will not show the patency of the ICA in its full extent in most patients, especially in those with weak

Table 1. Diagnostic criteria for grading of carotid artery stenosis

Diameter stenosis (category)	Peak systolic velocity (cm/sec)	Peak diastolic velocity (cm/sec)	Systolic velocity ratio (ICA/CCA)	Diastolic velocity ratio (ICA/CCA)
Grade 0 0%	<110	<40	<1.8	<2.4
Grade 1 1–39%	<110	<40	<1.8	<2.4
Grade 2 40–59%	<130	40	<1.8	<2.4
Grade 3 60–79%	>130	>40	>1.8	>2.4
Grade 4 80–99%	>250	>100	>3.7	>5.5

but still adequate collateral flow from the ECA to the carotid bifurcation or those with retrograde filling of the ICA by way of the Circle of Willis. Blackshear et al. and Keller et al. have used ultrasonic imaging of the carotid bifurcation by CW Doppler as well as duplex scanning to demonstrate the patency of the ICA and ECA distal to a common carotid occlusion. Nevertheless, these conventional methods are inadequate to detect the patency of the ICA reliably, because very reduced blood flow signals may not allow proper identification of the target artery. Flow direction in the ECA cannot be used as a reliable parameter since the artery may have a coiled or helical course. Application of CCDS in these cases provides an accurate determination of ICA patency in most instances. Since color imaging demonstrates a patent bifurcation quickly, both carotid branches can be shown and the fact that flow direction in the ECA is retrograde while ICA flow is antegrade (or possibly vice-versa) is readily appreciated; in most cases the ECA can be distinguished from the ICA by identification of ECA branches. The use of high sensitivity slow-flow settings makes it possible to assess even minimal blood flow in the ECA and ICA which is important since it prevents thrombus formation. The reliable diagnosis of a patent ICA by CCDS may be of therapeutic consequence for the patient.

Turbulence

Turbulence results in an increased range of flow velocities which leads to waveform changes known as spectral broadening in conventional Doppler systems. CCDS will display a mosaic pattern with a mixture of red and blue with different degrees of color saturation just distal to the stenosis (Fig. 50). This represents a combination of high-velocity areas, flow reversal, and aliasing. Color coding in real-time requires the simultaneous analysis of a high number of sample volumes. In contrast to duplex Doppler sonography, which gathers the flow information from only one sample volume and therefore offers enough time for a complete spectral analysis, color-Doppler imaging analyzes only the *mean* velocity in each sample volume and the variation from the mean of different velocities within the same sample volume.

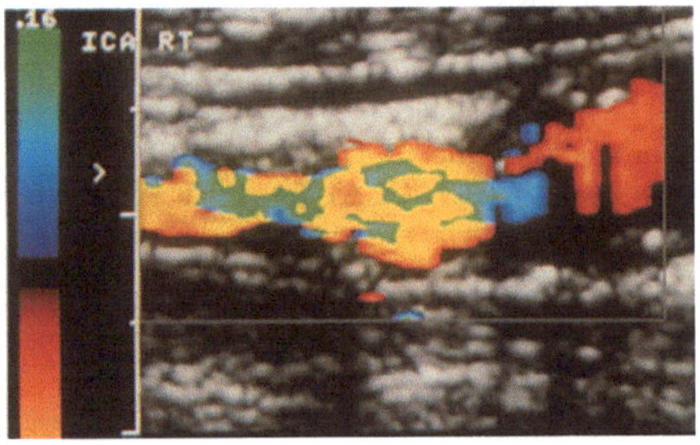

Fig. 50. Longitudinal sonogram of high-grade ICA stenosis with post-stenotic color mosaic pattern with a mixture of red and blue with different degrees of color saturation, indicating post-stenotic turbulence

The term "variance" is used to describe the degree to which velocities within a given sample volume differ from its mean velocity; variance can generally be thought to correspond to the amount of turbulent flow present. Color flow scanning units with special software (a velocity-variance program) have the ability to add additional color information (green is often used) in areas of significant flow disturbance; this enables a better delineation of turbulent areas and the separation of flow reversal zones and high-velocity areas (Figs. 51, 52). In the evaluation of patients with ICA stenoses greater than 50% it can be demonstrated that flow disturbances are maximal in the region immediately downstream from the stenosis; in the absence of additional areas of narrowing complete dissipation of the effects occur within 10 vessel diameters distally (Fig. 53). This observation correlates well with in vitro studies. Moreover, a direct correlation between the size of the region of disturbed flow and the degree of irregularity of the plaque surface within the stenosis can be shown. Distal to the stenosis there is an inverse relationship of the length of the region of flow disturbance to the *length* of the stenosis, and a direct relationship between length of the disturbed flow region and both the *grade* of the stenosis and the degree of plaque surface irregularity. In a few cases we noted turbulence exclusively within the area of stenosis without evidence of the generally expected post-stenotic component or significant pre-stenotic changes (Figs. 54, 55). Even

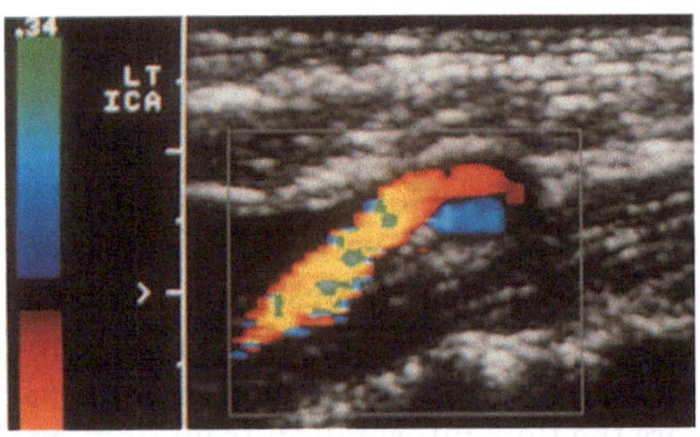

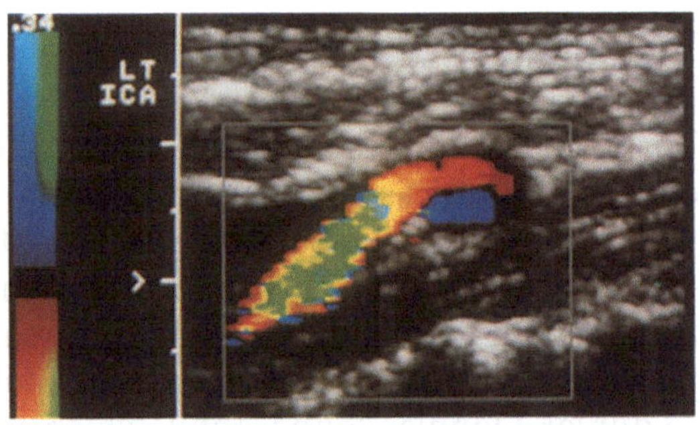

Figs. 51 (left), 52 (right). The same longitudinal sonogram of ICA with post-stenotic turbulence: comparison of routine color scale with velocity-variance program. The latter function adds additional color coding (green) in areas where velocity values differ significantly from the mean, resulting in better delineation of flow disturbance (turbulence)

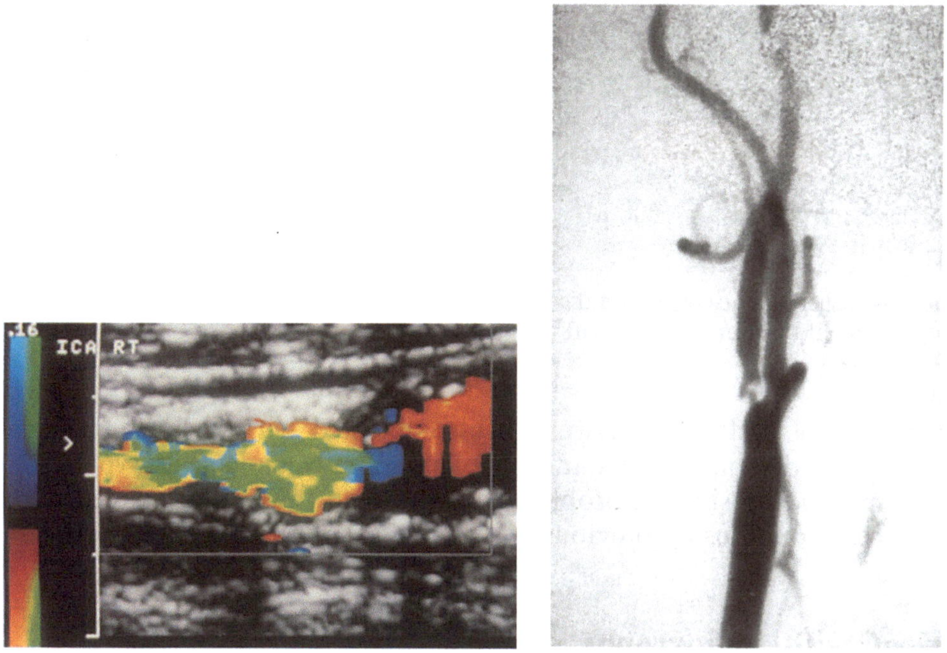

a b

Fig. 53. ***a*** Green-colored post-stenotic turbulent flow areas are shown extending several vessel diameters downstream; these changes are secondary to a short-segment, high-grade irregular stenosis at the ICA origin. ***b*** Angiography of same patient

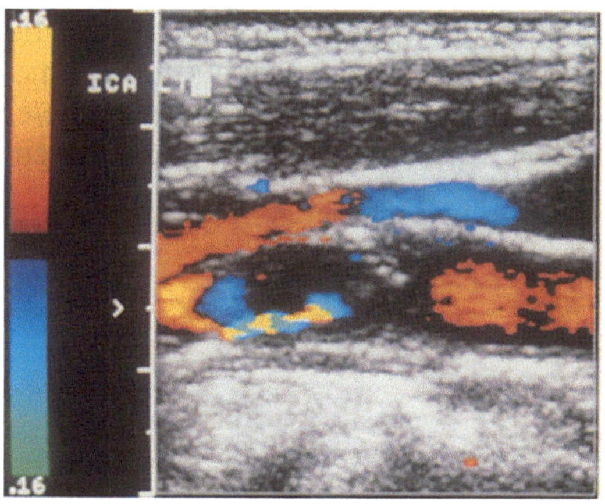

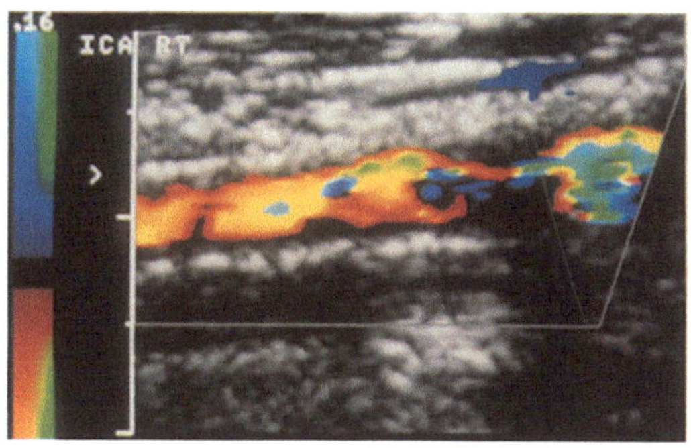

Fig. 54. (left) High-grade stenosis of ICA with intrastenotic green-coded turbulence but without evidence of post-stenotic turbulence

Fig. 55. (right) Filiform, short-segment ICA stenosis with turbulent flow, displayed in green color, *proximal* to the stenosis, but no significant post-stenotic turbulent areas

with high-grade stenosis there were some studies in which no related turbulent area could be identified. In patients with diameter reduction less than 50% a localized flow disturbance near the atheromatous plaque was shown in two-thirds of patients (Fig. 56). In the majority of these patients the region of disturbed flow could only be appreciated by use of the velocity-variance program. Application of color flow analysis with variance encoding may allow us to perform prospective studies on the

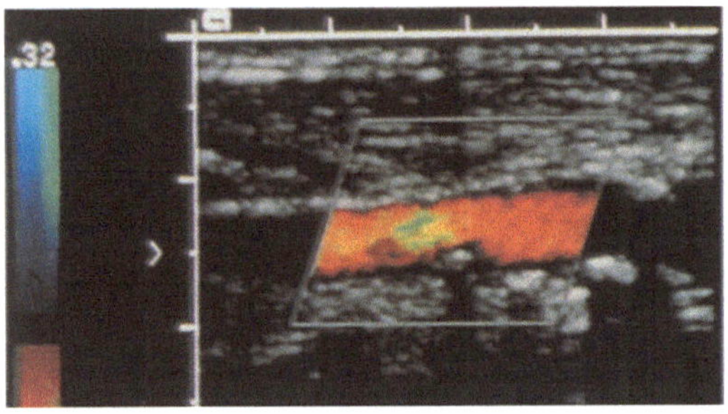

Fig. 56. Thornlike atheromatous plaque on the posterior CCA wall with a diameter reduction of less than 50% and regional turbulent flow (green)

characteristics of hemodynamic disturbances associated with various forms of carotid plaques to determine if separation of potentially dangerous types from benign ones may be possible (a problem for which no universally agreed-upon solution has been found using previously available sonographic techniques).

Comparison with angiography

Most authors cite angiography as the gold standard for the measurement of atherosclerotic stenosis in the ICA. Angiographic measurements, however, are imperfect for a number of reasons. First, prevalence of both intra- and inter-observer variability is 10–20%. Second, there is individual variability in the relative diameter of the carotid bulb in comparison with the more distal internal carotid artery. Angiographers have attempted to estimate the percent reduction in diameter directly by comparative measurement of the residual lumen and vessel diameter at the same level in the internal carotid artery (drawing 4). This measurement

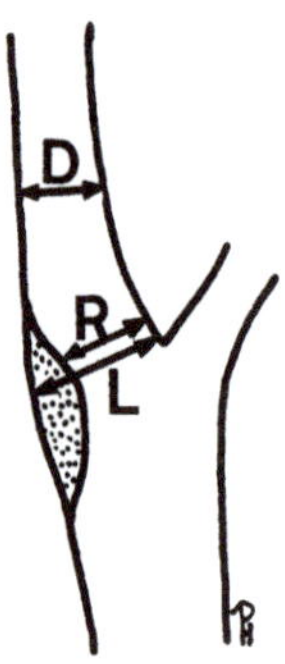

drawing 4

correlates best with the degree of stenosis, but it depends on an extrapolation of the pre- and post-stenotic segment of the artery, since the area outlined by contrast is no longer an accurate representation of true lumen diameter. Another approach is to determine arterial vessel diameter by noting wall calcifications (limited by the fact that wall calcification is not always present in diseased vessels). The more reproducible angiographic technique is to compare the diameter of the residual lumen at the site of greatest stenosis of the artery with the diameter of the more distal (and presumed normal) internal carotid artery. The presence of concentric distal plaque can result in an underestimation of the true distal internal carotid

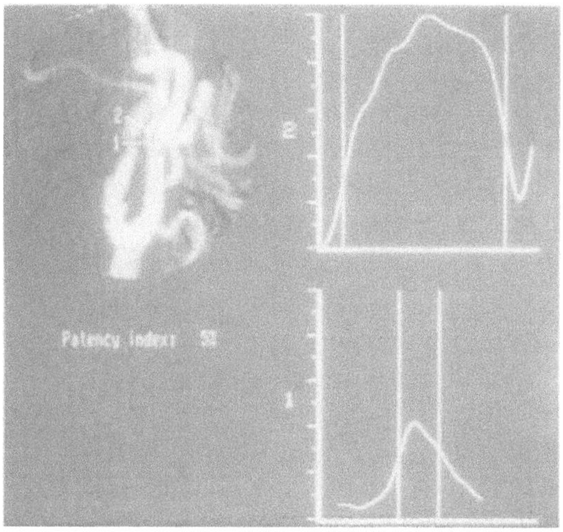

Fig. 57. Digital subtraction angiography (DSA): determination of a patency index

artery diameter resulting in a falsely low estimate of percentage of stenosis. Moreover, the individual variability of the carotid bulb is not taken into consideration; as a result, small to moderate plaques may go undetected. Another measurement technique is used with digital subtraction angiography: the density of the contrast medium at the area of maximal stenosis is compared to contrast density in a more distal non-stenotic segment of the artery and a patency index is derived. This method also has the disadvantage of depending on an individual definition of limits for measurement (Fig. 57). Other disadvantages of angiography include lack of images in the transverse plane and limitations as to definition of the morphology of the arterial wall; aortic arch angiograms alone may be inadequate for complete, accurate diagnosis.

ICA abnormalities associated with vessel enlargement

Because CCDS provides spatial display of Doppler frequency shift data from blood flow in vessels and organs which is superimposed on the B-mode image, it is a particularly useful technique for the demonstration of small-caliber vessels which would routinely go unnoticed during conventional duplex examination because of wall structure interference. This advantage of CCDS proves particularly useful in carotid body tumors where diagnosis is based on the easily recognized hypervascularity of the mass (Figs. 58, 59). Another diagnostic criterion is a widened contour of the bifurcation (Fig. 60). Demonstration of the increased vascularity is important in differentiating carotid body tumors from avascular or hypovascular cervical masses such as lymph node metastases, salivary gland tumors or (branchiogenic) cysts. CCDS provides only partial identification of the feeding arteries, so high-quality angiograms are still indicated before surgery.

In cases where cystic cervical lesions are noted in relationship to the internal carotid artery it has become accepted practice to make use of duplex Doppler to assess the mass for evidence of flow. But even if some portions of the lesion show evidence of abnormal flow it may still be difficult to differentiate between carotid

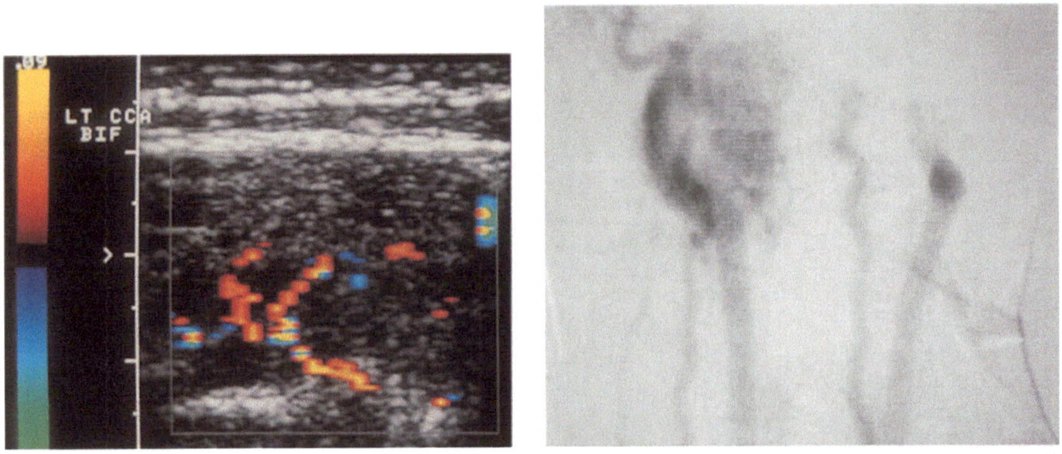

a *b*

Fig. 58. ***a*** CCDS shows a heterogeneous mass of low echogenicity containing multiple small-caliber vessels indicating hypervascularity (surgically proven carotid body tumor). ***b*** Intravenous angiogram of same patient

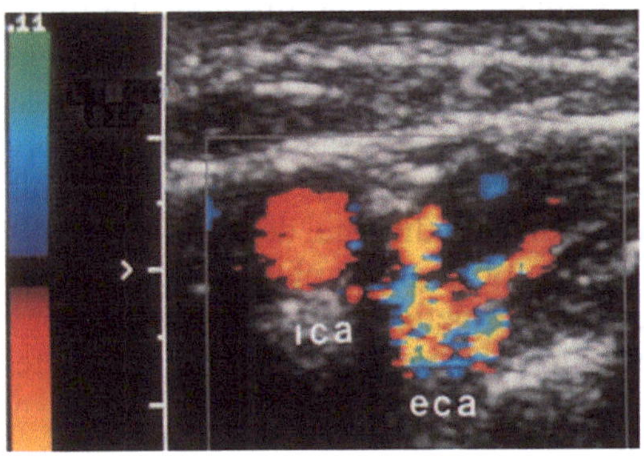

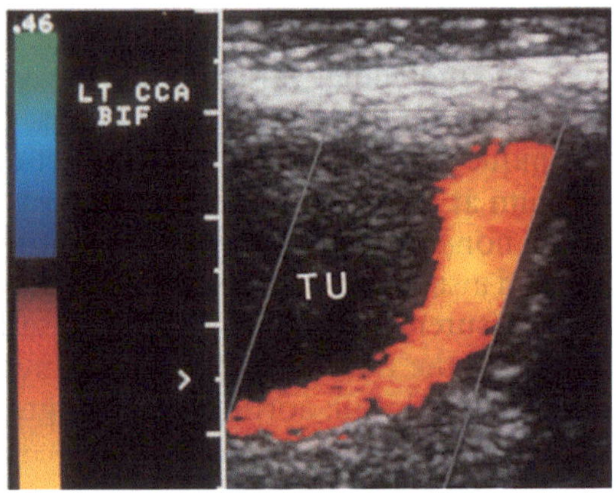

Fig. 59. (left) Transverse sonogram at the level of the carotid bifurcation shows tumor feeding vessels originating from the ECA

Fig. 60. (right) CCDS of a carotid body tumor demonstrates related ICA stretching and displacement

aneurysm and a tortuous course of the vessel. The addition of color flow mapping facilitates recognition of an aneurysm, where areas of absent flow may be shown to represent thrombotic material within a portion of the lumen. Using this approach it is possible to obtain adequate follow-up of patients after embolization (with balloons, for example) of a carotid aneurysm (Fig. 61). Prior to embolization, flow studies within the aneurysm demonstrate turbulent, high-velocity areas as well as slow-flow zones where there is a higher probability of thrombosis. After embolization the extent of thrombosis (or even complete occlusion) of the aneurysm can readily be assessed. In addition, the proximal and distal portions of the feeding artery can be evaluated with respect to their course and lumen diameter (Fig. 62).

The diagnosis of congenital or post-traumatic arteriovenous fistulas is easily established by conventional ultrasound and supplementary duplex Doppler evaluation. Additional information available with the use of CCDS includes subdivision of abnormally widened vessels into different categories: high velocity areas in the

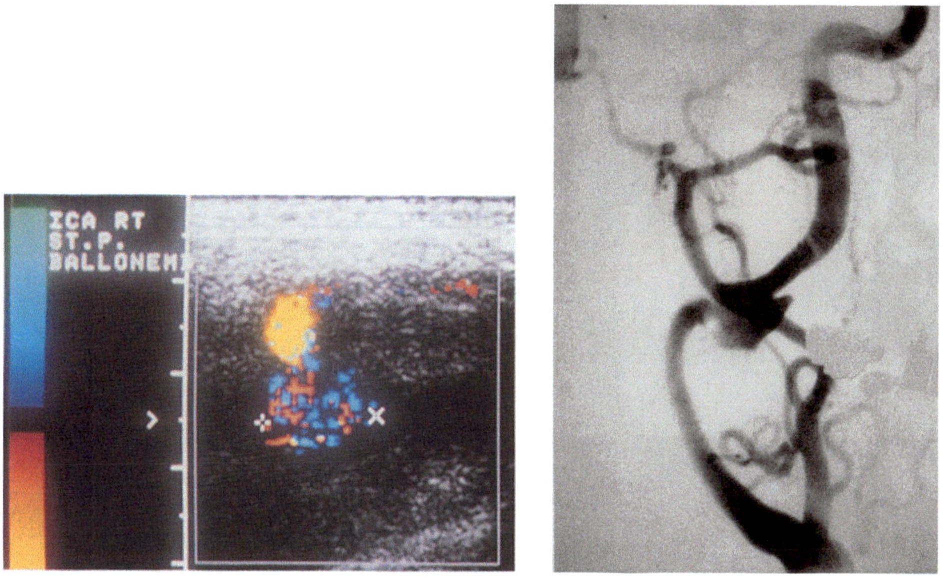

a *b*

Fig. 61. ***a*** CCDS of ICA aneurysm after interventional treatment with balloon embolization shows partial thrombosis with small patent lumen in its cranial portion. ***b*** Angiogram of same patient

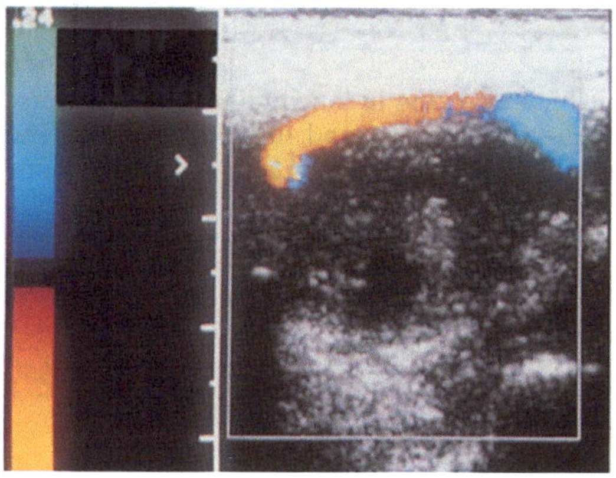

Fig. 62. Ventral displacement and moderate narrowing of the ICA due to the thrombosed aneurysm

region of direct arterial-to-venous shunting, which are identified by jet phenomena and turbulence; and slow-flow zones (for which slow-flow sensitivity settings must be employed) which are of importance in selecting patients for embolization therapy since areas of slow flow increase the probability of successful thrombosis (Figs. 63, 64). This categorization is not possible on the basis of angiographic findings. This hypothesis regarding noninvasive evaluation of A-V fistulas needs further assessment by a larger number of treated patients. CCDS also allows assessment of which cervical vessels are involved in formation of the fistula complex since the area surrounding the fistula can be readily seen (Fig. 65). Supplying arteries from the ICA, thyrocervical trunk, subclavian artery and even the vertebral artery can be identified. High quality selective angiograms are still necessary prior to interventional therapy or surgery.

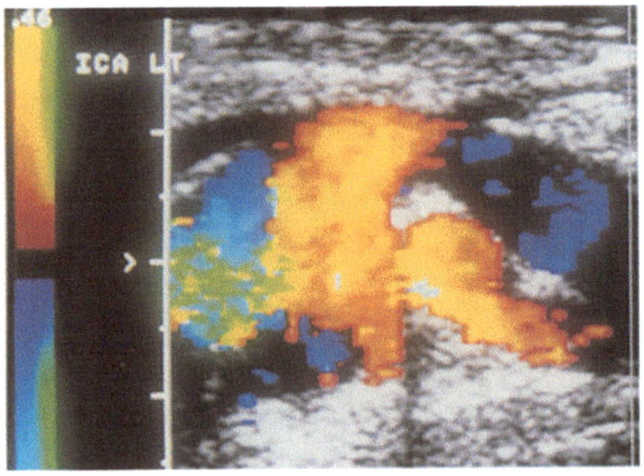

63

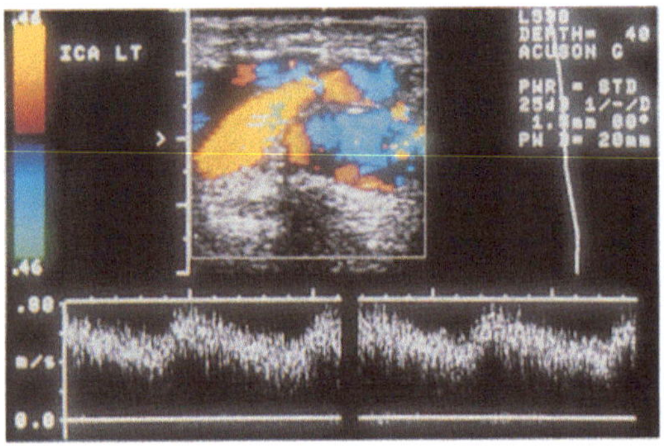

64 a

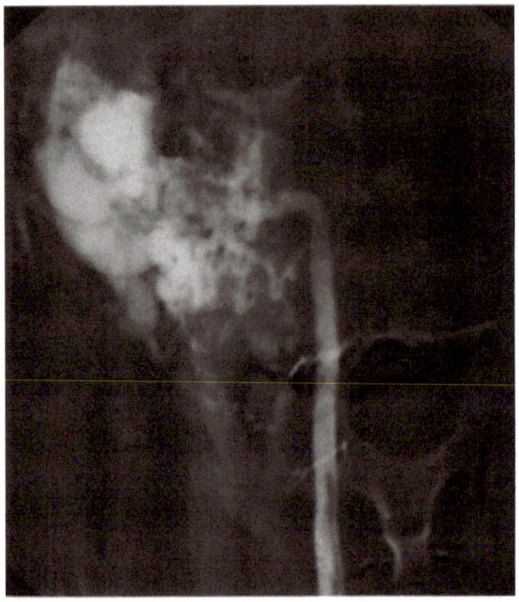

64 b

Figs. 63, 64 ***a***. CCDS of carotid artery arterio-venous malformation in longitudinal and transverse planes shows multiple abnormal widened vessels, high-velocity areas, and turbulent regions. The spectral tracing demonstrates characteristic high diastolic flow velocities. 64 ***b*** Angiogram of same patient

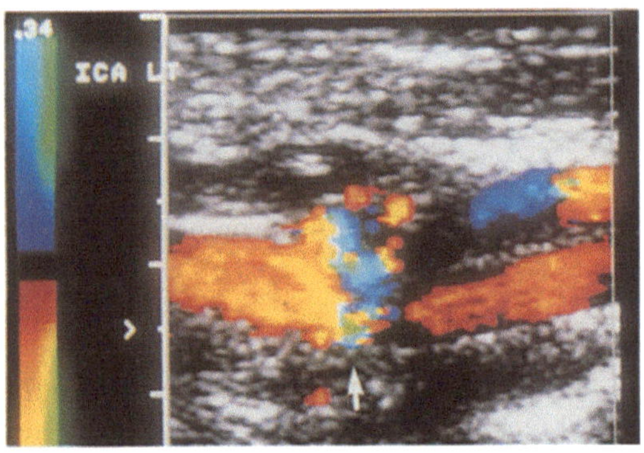

Fig. 65. Longitudinal CCDS image demonstrates an arterio-venous fistula from the ICA with jet-phenomenon and (green) turbulent flow (arrow)

In practice, color flow imaging allows the sonographer to scan the carotid artery quickly in transverse section and to identify the region of its bifurcation and the direction taken by the internal and external carotids. This is especially helpful if there is tortuosity of the vessels (Figs. 66, 67). In marked coiling of the ICA, differentiation from an aneurysm without thrombosis may be difficult; CCDS allows an exact delineation of vessel course and the evaluation of hemodynamics

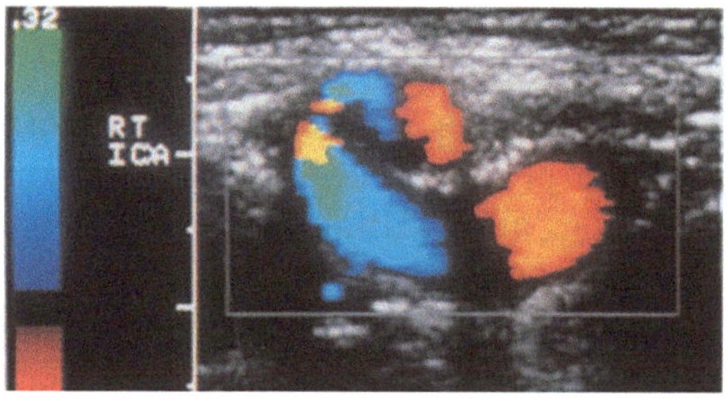

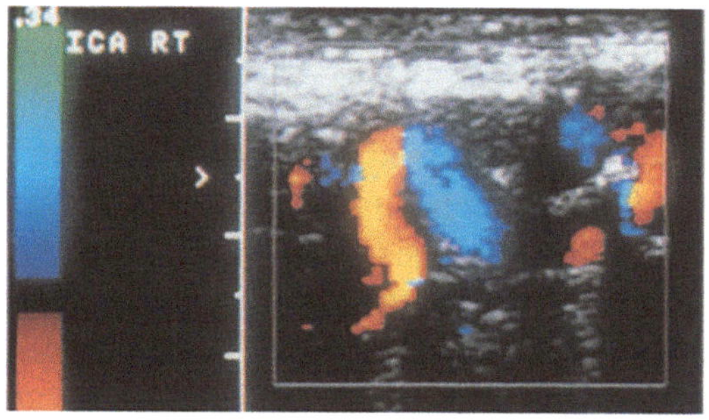

Fig. 66. (left) CCDS of ICA tortuosity with a 360° loop and distinct change of color because of different flow directions with respect to the transducer

Fig. 67. (right) Longitudinal CCDS view of ICA demonstrates a 180° kinking of the vessel without significant lumen diameter reduction

along the vessel, particularly the identification of associated stenotic segments. In patients with demonstrated kinking or coiling in one carotid vessel it is often possible to show similar changes of the contralateral carotid or in the vertebral arteries (see vertebral artery chapter).

Carotid artery dissection may occur spontaneously but is more commonly due to extension from a dissection originally involving the aorta. CCDS allows identification of carotid dissection with evaluation of possible extension from the CCA to the ICA and assessment of direction of flow in both lumens. The detection of even slow-flowing blood in the false lumen by CCDS will avoid misdiagnosis of thrombosis. Conversely, absence of color-coding in a false lumen even at high sensitivity settings indicates that thrombosis has occurred. With conventional duplex sonography a duplication ("mirror") artifact from the deep wall of the common carotid artery may lead to a misdiagnosis of a patent false lumen.

Postoperative examination

It has been shown that a hemodynamically significant decrease in flow to the brain does not occur until narrowing of the carotid artery exceeds 75% of the cross-sectional area or 50% of the diameter. In patients with TIA symptoms and stenosis exceeding these values in the extracranial carotid artery it has been thought that carotid endarterectomy may be of benefit. This impression is supported by a recent report from the North American Symptomatic Carotid Endarterectomy Trial Collaboration (New England Journal of Medicine, August 15, 1991, 445–453) which concluded that "Carotid endarterectomy is highly beneficial to patients with recent hemispheric and retinal transient ischemic attacks or nondisabling strokes and ipsilateral high-grade stenosis (70 to 99 percent) of the internal carotid artery". Following endarterectomy the sonographic appearance of the carotid is identical to that of a normal carotid artery except that there will be no intimal echoes within the area of surgery, and the walls may appear ectatic or dilated. There may be a distinct "shelf" of intimal lining in the distal common carotid artery, which marks the lower point of the endarterectomy. Flow dynamics with CCDS and direct Doppler assessment will be much the same as in the normal examination with one exception: because of decreased resistance and an increase in the elasticity of the carotid wall in the endarterectomy area, large flow reversal zones may be seen. This will be more pronounced if a saphenous vein patch has been used. In the literature restenosis of the ICA after thrombendarterectomy is reported in 8.8% to 36% of cases (excluding acute thrombosis in the postoperative period). Patients with *symptomatic* restenosis comprise a smaller group of 1.5 to 4.8%. Two different types of restenosis can be distinguished pathologically: within 24 months after surgery myointimal hyperplasia may occur; later-developing restenoses are due to recurrent atheromatous plaque formation. In a series of 51 patients who had undergone a total of 64 carotid thrombendarterectomies, follow-up by duplex sonography identified five asymptomatic occlusions of the ICA (8%) and one occlusion of the CCA. Two patients (3%) developed a restenosis of more than 50% and another two patients a restenosis of less than 50%. Changes in the vessel wall not producing significant luminal change were observed in another 18 cases (28%). Thirty-six of the operated vessels (56%) showed no change. In a long-term noninvasive follow-up after carotid endarterectomy (248 arteries) the absolute incidence of recurrent carotid disease was 28% with a 13% incidence of hemodynamically significant restenosis and a 15% incidence of hemodynamically insignificant disease. The incidence of ipsilateral neurologic events was 8%.

CCDS is also helpful in the post-operative evaluation of surgically created extracranial-to-intracranial shunts, such as a superficial temporal artery to middle cerebral artery bypass (Figs. 68, 69, 70). Patency, areas of focal stenosis, and significant changes over time during follow-up can all be well evaluated noninvasively.

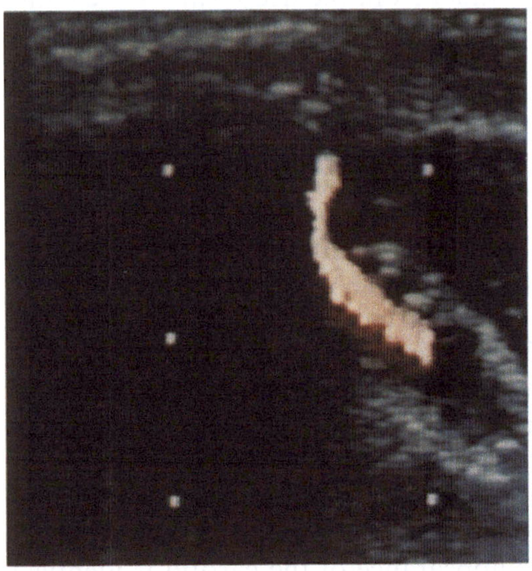

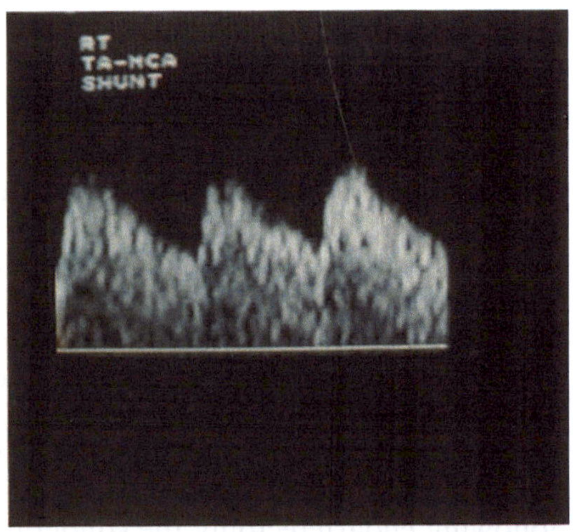

Fig. 68. (left) CCDS of right superficial temporal artery to middle cerebral artery shunt in an 8 year old girl with a history of bilateral ICA occlusions secondary to moyamoya disease. The ability to confirm the patency of her (bilateral) shunts noninvasively has been particularly significant because of a pronounced tendency to vasospasm whenever arteriography has been attempted in the past

Fig. 69. (right) Spectral waveform tracing from superficial temporal artery to middle cerebral artery shunt (same case as Fig. 68) showing high diastolic flow (low-resistance pattern) typical of vessels supplying the intracranial vascular bed

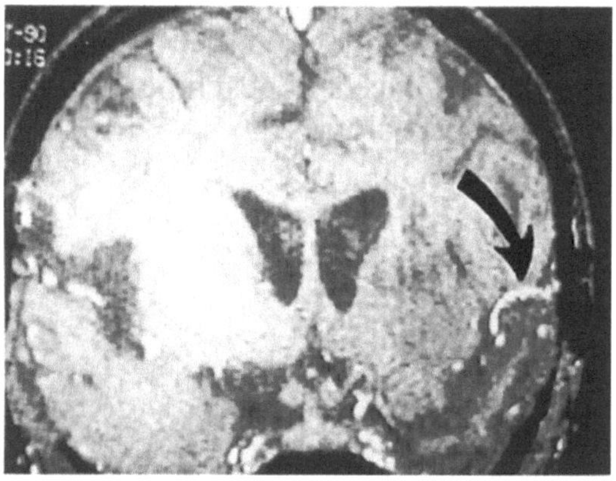

Fig. 70. Magnetic resonance angiogram showing patency of left superficial temporal artery to middle cerebral artery shunt (curved arrow; same case as Figs. 68, 69); the right shunt is partially visualized as well

In view of all the advantages noted above, color-coded Doppler sonography is now the method of choice for noninvasive follow-up of patients following carotid endarterectomy or extracranial-to-intracranial shunting procedures.

Summary

CCDS not only preserves the documented advantages of conventional sonography and duplex sonography but also provides important additional diagnostic information. Examples include better differentiation of smooth and irregular surface structures and identification of ulcerative niches, both of which may be underlying causes of embolic cerebrovascular events; better assessment of anechoic plaque components such as necrotic and thrombotic material by absence of the color flow signal; and visualization of hemodynamic disturbances associated with various plaque configurations, giving us a tool for prospective studies which should lead to a better understanding of the pathogenesis of ischemic cerebral events. Considering these advantages, CCDS is superior to angiography, previously considered the "gold standard", in the evaluation of extracranial carotid artery disease. Moreover, grading of stenosis by CCDS is preferable to angiography-based grading because of the ability to obtain transverse images as well as more accurate demonstration of the true luminal diameter at the same level as the stenosis. As a consequence, the majority of patients with high-grade carotid artery stenosis and ipsilateral symptoms may now go directly to endarterectomy without angiography, at least in centers where the surgeons have a high level of confidence in the ultrasound diagnostic information available to them. CCDS is able to provide accurate information even in the presence of tortuous vessels, an area of weakness for conventional duplex Doppler examination. Difficulties remain even for CCDS, however, in the presence of a high location of the carotid bifurcation, where adequate visualization of the proximal portions of the ICA and ECA may be difficult. When large calcified plaques are present, distal acoustic shadowing may preclude adequate color imaging; this limitation may be somewhat overcome by careful evaluation of the pre- and post-stenotic portions of the vessel. Postoperative examinations are now routinely performed using CCDS. When compared with conventional duplex sonography CCDS allows shorter examination times, facilitates interpretation of even complex findings, and serves as an excellent teaching tool for familiarizing residents with vascular anatomy and pathology.

References

Adachi B (1928) Das Arteriensystem der Japaner. In: Adachi B (Hrsg) Anatomie der Japaner, Bd 1, 1. Aufl. Verlag der Kaiserlich-Japanischen Universität zu Kyoto, Kyoto

Barnett HJM (1978) Delayed cerebral ischemic episodes distal to occlusion of major cerebral arteries. Neurology 28:769–774

Barnett HJM, Peerless SJ, Kaufmann JCM (1978) "Stump" of internal carotid artery – a source for further cerebral embolic ischemia. Stroke 9:448–456

Beckett WW, Davis PC, Hoffman JC Jr (1990) Duplex Doppler sonography of the carotid artery: False-positive results in an artery contralateral to an artery with marked stenosis. AJR 155: 1090–1095

Beneficial effect of carotid endarterectomy in symptomatic patients with high-grade carotid stenosis (1991) Report from the North American Symptomatic Carotid Endarterectomy Trial Collaborators. N Engl J Med 325:445–453

Bharadvaj BK, Mabon RF, Giddens DP (1982a) Steady flow in a model of the human bifurcation. Part I: Flow visualization. J Biomech 15:349–362

Bharadvaj BK, Mabon RF, Giddens DP (1982b) Steady flow in a model of human bifurcation. Part II: Laser – Doppler anemometer measurements. J Biomech 15:363–378

Blackshear WM Jr, Phillips DJ, Bodily KC, Strandness DE Jr (1980) Ultrasonic demonstration of external and internal carotid patency with common carotid occlusion: a preliminary report. Stroke 3:249–252

Blackwell E, Merory J, Toole JF, McKinney WM (1977) Doppler ultrasound scanning of the carotid bifurcation. Arch Neurol 34:145–148

Blackwell DE, McKinney WM, Nunn C, Hirsch G, Sackler JP (1984) Low cost real-time Doppler frequency analysis. Medical Ultrasound 8:23–29

Blaisdell WF, Clauss RH, Galbraith JG, Imparato AM, Wylie EJ (1969) Joint study of extracranial arterial occlusion. IV. A review of surgical considerations. JAMA 209

Blue SK, McKinney WM, Barnes R, Toole JF (1972) Ultrasonic B-mode scanning for study of extracranial vascular disease. Neurology 22:1081–1085

Bluth EI, Shyn PB, Sullivan MA, Merritt ChRB (1989) Doppler flow imaging of carotid artery dissection. J Ultrasound Med 8:149–153

Bluth EI, Stavros AT, Marich KW, Wetzner SM, Aufrichtig D, Baker JD (1988) Carotid duplex sonography: A multicenter recommendation for standardized imaging and Doppler criteria. Radiographics 3

Bo WJ, McKinney WM, Bowden RL (1989) The origin and distribution of vasa vasorum at the bifurcation of the common carotid artery with atherosclerosis. Stroke 20:1484–1487

Breslau PJ, Knox RA, Phillips DJ, Beach KW, Chikos PM, Thiele BL, Strandness DE Jr (1982) Ultrasonic duplex scanning with spectral analysis in extracranial carotid artery disease. Vascular Diag Therapy 3:17–22

Brown MS, Kovanen PT, Goldstein JL (1981) Regulation of plasma cholesterol by lipoprotein receptors. Science 212:628–635

Brown PB, Zwiebel WJ, Call GK (1989) Degree of cervical carotid artery stenosis and hemispheric stroke: Duplex US findings. Radiology 170:541–543

Cisneros JA, Newhouse VL, Goldberg B (1985) Doppler spectral characterization of flow disturbances in the carotid with the Doppler probe at right angles to the vessel axis. Ultrasound Med Biol 11:319–328

Clagett GP, Patterson CB, Fisher DF Jr, Fry RE, Eidt JF, Humble TH, Fry WJ (1989) Vein patch versus primary closure for carotid endarterectomy. A randomized prospective study in a selected group of patients. J Vasc Surg 9(2):213–223

Craven TE, Ryu JE, Espeland MA, Kahl FR, McKinney WM, Toole JF, et al (1990) Evaluation of the association between carotid artery atherosclerosis and coronary artery stenosis. A case-control study. Circulation 82:1230–1242
Crissey MM, Bernstein EF (1974) Delayed presentation of carotid intimal tear following blunt craniocervical trauma. Surgery 75:543–549
Crouse JR, Toole JF, McKinney WM, Dignan MB, Howard G, Kahl FR, McMahan MR, Harpold GH (1987) Risk factors for extracranial carotid artery atherosclerosis. Stroke 6:990–996
Crowe WJ, Krovetz LJ (1972) Studies of arterial branching in models using flow birefringence. Med Biol Engng 10:415–426
DeGroote RD, Lynch TG, Jamil Z, Hobson RW (1987) Carotid restenosis: long-term noninvasive follow-up after carotid endarterectomy. Stroke 18:1031–1036
Douville Y, Johnston KW, Kassam M (1985) Determination of the hemodynamic factors which influence carotid Doppler spectral broadening. Ultrasound Med Biol 11:417–423
Dyken ML, Klatte E, Kolar OJ, Surgeon C (1974) Complete occlusion of common or internal carotid arteries. Clinical significance. Arch Neurol 30:343–346
Eckmann A, Kuhn FP, Grönniger J (1986) Postoperative Verlaufskontrolle der A. carotis mit der Duplex-Sonographie. Fortschr Röntgenstr 145:639–641
Erickson SJ, Newissen MW, Foley WD, Lawson TL, Middleton WD, Quiroz FA, Macrander SJ, Lipchik EO (1989) Stenosis of the internal carotid artery: assessment using color Doppler imaging compared with angiography. AJR 152:1299–1305
Fei DY, Billian C, Rittgers SE (1988) Flow dynamics in a stenosed carotid bifurcation model – Part I: Basic velocity measurements. Ultrasound Med Biol 14:21–31
Fell G, Phillips DJ, Chikos PM, Harley JD, Thiele BL, Strandness DE Jr (1981) Ultrasonic duplex scanning for disease of the carotid artery. Circulation 64:1191–1195
Födisch HJ (1970) Die Thrombosen der A. carotis und ihrer Äste nach stumpfen Traumen. In: Löhr B, Senning A, Witt AN (Hrsg) Ergebnisse der Chirurgie und Orthopädie 53:75–98
Fox JA, Hugh AE (1966) Localization of atheroma: A theory based on boundary layer separation. Br Heart J 28:388–399
Genton E, Barnett HJM, Fields WS, Gent M, Hoak JC (1977) Report of the joint committee for stroke resources XIV: Cerebral ischemia, the role of thrombosis and antithrombotic therapy. Stroke 8:147–175
Giddens DP, Mabon RF, Cassanova RA (1976) Measurements of disordered flow distal to subtotal vascular stenoses in the thoracic aortas of dogs. Circ Res 39:112–119
Glover JL, Bendick PJ, Dilly RS, Jackson VP, Reilly MK, Dalsing MC, Robison RJ (1985) Restenosis following carotid endarterectomy. Arch Surg 120:678–683
Glover JL, Bendick PJ, Jackson VP, Becker GJ, Dilley RS, Holden RW (1984) Duplex ultrasonography, digital subtraction angiography and conventional angiography in assessing carotid atherosclerosis. Arch Surg 119:664–669
Hallam MJ, Reid J, Cooperberg PL (1989) Color-flow Doppler and conventional Duplex scanning of the carotid bifurcation: Prospective, double-blind, correlative study. AJR 152:1101–1105
Hass WK, Fields WS, North RR, Kricheff H, Chase NE, Bauer RB (1968) Joint study of extracranial arterial occlusion. II. Arteriography, techniques, sites, and complications. JAMA 203:159–166
Hennerici M, Freund HJ (1984) Efficacy of CW-Doppler and duplex system examinations for the evaluation of extracranial carotid disease. JCU 12:155–161
Hertzer NR, Flanagan RA, O'Hara PJ, Beven EG (1986) Surgical versus nonoperative treatment of asymptomatic carotid stenosis. Ann Surg 204:163–171
Houi K, Mochio S, Isogai Y, Miyamoto Y, Suzuki N (1990) Comparison of color flow and 3D image by computer graphics for the evaluation of carotid disease. Angiology 41(4):305–312
Hübsch P, Schwaighofer B, Karnel F, Braunsteiner A, Frühwald F, Pichler W, Trattnig S (1988) Farbcodierte Dopplersonographie der Karotiden. Röntgen Fortschr 149:189–192
Hutchison KJ, Karpinski E (1985) In vivo demonstration of flow recirculation and turbulence downstream of graded stenoses in canine arteries. J Biomech 18:285–296
Imparato AM, Riles TS, Gorstein F (1979) The carotid bifurcation plaque: pathologic findings associated with cerebral ischemia. Stroke 10:238–245
Jacobs NM, Grant EG, Schellinger D, Byrd MC, Richardson JD, Cohan SL (1985) Duplex carotid sonography: Criteria for stenosis, accuracy, and pitfalls. Radiology 154:385–391
Javid H, Ostermiller WE, Hengesh JW, Dye WS, Hunter JA, Najafi H, Julian OC (1970) Natural history of carotid bifurcation atheroma. Surgery 67:80–86

Kalman PG, Johnston KW, Zuech P, Kassam M, Potts K (1985) In vitro comparison of alternative methods for quantifying the severity of Doppler spectral broadening for the diagnosis of carotid arterial occlusive disease. Ultrasound Med Biol 11:435–440
Kassam M, Johnston KW, Cobbold RSC (1985) Quantitative estimation of spectral broadening for the diagnosis of carotid arterial disease: Method and in vitro results. Ultrasound Med Biol 11: 425–433
Keller HM, Valavanis A, Imhof HG, Turina M (1984) Patency of external and internal carotid artery in the presence of an occluded common carotid artery: Noninvasive evaluation with combined cerebrovascular Doppler examination and sequential computertomography. Stroke 1:149–157
Khalifa AMA, Giddens DP (1981) Characterization and evolution of post-stenotic flow disturbances. J Biomech 14:279–296
Lapayowker MS, Stauffer HM, Safer JN (1972) Physiologic stasis of roentgenographic contrast material at the carotid artery bifurcation: Possible correlation to atheroma localization. Am J Roentgenol Radium Therm Nucl Med 114:803–809
Lechner H, Niederkorn K, Suzuki H (1987) Hemorrheologic parameters in correlation to extracranial carotid disease in patients with acute cerebrovascular disorders. Eur Neurol 27:139–141
Lewis BD, James EM, Charboneau JW, Reading CC, Welch TJ (1989) Current applications of color Doppler imaging in the abdomen and extremities. Radiographics 4
Liou RJ, Clark ME, Robertson JM (1981) Three-dimensional simulation of steady flow past a partial stenosis. J Biomech 14:325–337
Londrey GL, Spadone DP, Hodgson KJ, Ramsey DE, Barkmeier LD, Sumner GS (1991) Does color-flow imaging improve the accuracy of duplex carotid evaluation? J Vasc Surg 13(5):569–663
Lo LY, Ford CS, McKinney WM, Toole JF (1986) Asymptomatic bruit, carotid and vertebrobasilar transient ischemic attacks – a clinical and ultrasonic correlation. Stroke 17:65–68
Lusby RJ, Ferrell LD, Ehrenfeld WK, et al. (1982) Carotid plaque hemorrhage: its role in production of cerebral ischemia. Arch Surg 117:1479–1488
Lutz RJ, Hsu L, Menawat A, Zrubek J, Edwards K (1983) Comparison of steady and pulsatile flow in a double branching arterial model. J Biomech 16:753–766
Lynch PR, Bonakdarpour A, Stauffer HM, Heckman JL (1973) Angiographic evidence of stagnant flow zones in the carotid circulation of anesthetized dogs. Invest Radiol 8:28–32
Malcolm AD, Roach MR (1979) Flow disturbances at the apex and lateral angles of a variety of bifurcation models and their role in development and manifestations of arterial disease. Stroke 10:335–343
Mattle HP, Kent KC, Edelman RR, Atkinson DJ, Skillman JJ (1991) Evaluation of the extracranial carotid arteries: correlation of magnetic resonance angiography, duplex ultrasonography, and conventional angiography. J Vasc Surg 13:838–844, discussion 844–845
Middleton WD, Foley WD, Lawson TL (1988) Color-flow Doppler imaging of carotid abnormalities. AJR 150:419–425
Middleton WD, Foley WD, Lawson TL (1988) Flow reversal in the normal carotid bifurcation: Color Doppler flow imaging analysis. Radiology 167:207–210
Middleton WD, Melson GL (1990) The carotid ghost: A color Doppler ultrasound duplication artifact. J Ultrasound Med 9:487–493
Moore DJ, Sheehan MP, Kolm MS, Russell JB, Sumner DS (1985) Are strokes predictable with noninvasive methods: a five-year follow up of 303 unoperated patients. J Vasc Surg 2:654–660
Motomiya M, Karino Takeshi (1984) Flow patterns in the human carotid artery bifurcation. Stroke 1:50–56
Niederkorn K, Horner S, Schmidt R, Fazekas F, Lechner H (1991) Ultrasonic assessment of the prevalence of carotid artery stenosis in asymptomatic volunteers. J Neuroimaging 1:119–122
Nicholls SC, Phillips DJ, Primozich JF, Lawrence RL, Kohler TR, Rudd TG, Strandness DE Jr (1989) Diagnostic significance of flow separation in the carotid bulb. Stroke 20:175–182
O'Brien V, Ehrlich LW (1985) Simple pulsatile flow in an artery with a constriction. J Biomech 18: 117–127
O'Donnell TF Jr, Erdoes L, Mackey WC, et al. (1985) Correlation of B-mode ultrasound imaging and arteriography with pathologic findings of carotid endarterectomy. Arch Surg 120:443–449
Palmaz JC, Hunter G, Carson SN, French SW (1983) Postoperative carotid restenosis due to neointimal fibromuscular hyperplasia. Radiology 148:669–702
Podore PC, Rob CG, DeWeese JA, Green RM (1981) Chronic common carotid artery occlusion. Stroke 12:98–100

Polak JF, Dobkin GR, O'Leary DH, Wang AM, Cutler SS (1989) Internal carotid artery stenosis: Accuracy and reproducibility of color-Doppler-assisted duplex imaging. Radiology 173(3): 793–798

Quill DS, Colgan MP, Sumner DS (1989) Carotid stump syndrome: a colour-coded Doppler flow study. Eur J Vasc Surg 3:79–83

Rayman R, Kratky RG, Roach MR (1985) Steady flow visualization in a rigid canine aortic cast. J Biomech 18:863–875

Reilly LM, Lusby RJ, Hughes L, Ferrell LD, Stoney RJ, Ehrenfeld WK (1983) Carotid plaque histology using real-time ultrasonography: clinical and therapeutic implications. Am J Surg 146:188–193

Rittgers SE, Fei DY (1988) Flow dynamics in a stenosed carotid bifurcation model – Part II: Derived indices. Ultrasound Med Biol 14

Rittgers SE, Thornhill BM, Barnes RW (1983) Quantitative analysis of carotid artery Doppler spectral waveforms: Diagnostic value of parameters. Ultrasound Med Biol 9:255–264

Robinson ML, Sacks D, Perlmutter GS, Marinelli DL (1988) Diagnostic criteria for carotid duplex sonography. AJR 151:487–506

Roederer GO, Langlois YE, Jager KA (1984) The natural history of carotid arterial disease in asymptomatic patients with cervical bruits. Stroke 15:605–613

Schwaighofer BW, Trattnig S (1990) Farbkodierte Dopplersonographie der Arteria carotis. Radiologe 30:511–515

Sheldon CD, Murie JA, Quin RO (1983) Ultrasonic Doppler spectral broadening in the diagnosis of internal carotid artery stenosis. Ultrasound Med Biol 9:575–580

Shulak JM, O'Donovan PB, Paushter DM, Lanzieri CF (1989) Color flow Doppler of carotid body paraganglioma. J Ultrasound Med 8(9):519–521

Siouffi M, Pellisier R, Farahifar D, Rieu R (1984) The effect of unsteadiness of flow through stenoses and bifurcations. J Biomech 17:299–315

So EL, Toole JF, Moody DM, Challa VR (1979) Cerebral embolism from septal fibromuscular dysplasia of the common carotid artery. Ann Neurol 6:75–78

Steinke W, Hennerici M, Aulich A (1988) Doppler Color flow imaging of carotid body tumors. Stroke 11:1574–1577

Steinke W, Kloetzsch Ch, Hennerici M (1990) Carotid artery disease assessed by color Doppler flow imaging: Correlation with standard Doppler sonography and angiography. Am J Roentgenol 154 (5):1061–1068

Sterpetti AV, Schultz RD, Feldhaus RJ, Davenport KL, Richardson M, Farina C, Hunter WJ (1988) Ultrasonographic features of carotid plaque and the risk of subsequent neurologic deficits. Surgery 104:652–660

Sumner DS (1990) Use of color-flow imaging technique in carotid artery disease (Review Article – 17 references). Surg Clin North Am 70(1):201–211

Tell GS, Howard G, McKinney WM, Toole JF (1989) Cigarette smoking cessation and extracranial carotid atherosclerosis. JAMA 261:1178–1180

Terwey B, Gahbauer H, Montemayor M, Proussalis A, Zöllner G (1984) Die B-Bild-Sonographie der Karotisbifurkation. Ultraschall 5:190–201

Trattnig S, Hübsch P, Barton P, Karnel F, Sautner Th, Schwaighofer B, Kretschmer G (1991) Durchgängigkeit der Karotis externa und interna bei Patienten mit Karotis communis Okklusion: Nachweis in der farbkodierten Dopplersonographie. Fortschr Röntgenstr 154:44–48

Trattnig S, Schwaighofer B, Hübsch P, Kainberger F, Pölzleitner D (1990) Velocity-Variance-Funktion. Zusatzinformation in der farbkodierten Dopplersonographie der Karotiden. Fortschr Röntgenstr 153:663–668

Trattnig S, Schwaighofer B, Kainberger F, Hübsch P (1990) Flußumkehr in der Karotisbifurkation. Nachweis in der farbkodierten Doppler-Sonographie. Radiologe 30:516–519

Weibel J, Fields WS (1969) Atlas of arteriography in occlusive cerebrovascular disease. Georg Thieme, Stuttgart

Weinberger J, Marks SJ, Gaul JJ, Goldman B, Schanzer H, Jacobson J, Dikman S (1987) Atherosclerotic plaque at the carotid artery bifurcation: Correlation of ultrasonographic imaging with morphology. J Ultrasound Med 6:363–366

Widder B, von Reutern GM, Neuerburg-Heusler D (1986) Morphologische und Dopplersonographische Kriterien zur Bestimmung von Stenosierungsgraden an der A. carotis interna. Ultraschall 7:70–75

Wilhelmson L, Svardsudd K, Korsan-Bengsten K, et al (1984) Fibrinogen as a risk factor for stroke and myocardial infarction. N Engl J Med 311: 501–505

Wylie J, Effency DJ (1979) Surgery of aortic arch branches and vertebral artery. Surg Clin North Am 59: 669–680

Zarins CK, Giddens DP, Bharadvaj BK, Sottiurai VS, Mabon RF, Glagov S (1983) Carotid bifurcation atherosclerosis: Quantitative correlation of plaque localization with flow velocity profiles and wall shear stress. Circ Res 53: 502–514

Zwiebel WJ, Austin CW, Sackett JF, Strother CM (1983) Correlation of high-resolution B-mode and continuous-wave Doppler sonography with arteriography in the diagnosis of carotid stenosis. Radiology 149: 523–532

Zwicker C, Langer M, Mäurer J, Hepp W (1986) Angiomorphologie arteriosklerotischer Gefäßveränderungen im Bereich der Karotisbifurkation. Röntgenblätter 39: 209–215

4 Color-coded Doppler sonography of the vertebral arteries

S. Trattnig, P. Hübsch, and F. Frühwald

Introduction

The common carotid artery and the origins of the internal and external carotid arteries are relatively superficial in the anterolateral portion of the neck, making them readily accessible for direct examination by noninvasive techniques. This is not the case with the vertebral arteries, which are more deeply placed in the neck; in their midcervical course they are largely obscured by bone as they pass through the transverse processes of C6-C2. For this reason, Doppler vertebral examination is subject to difficulties and limitations not encountered in carotid studies.

For many years continuous wave Doppler sonography was the most important tool for the non-invasive investigation of the extracranial vertebral arteries. With this technique the vertebral arteries could not be visualized and vessel identification was often difficult. The introduction of duplex Doppler systems made vessel visualization possible and provided the capability for evaluation of flow characteristics in different segments of the vertebral arteries. With color-coded Doppler sonography (CCDS) we now have access to immediate information about blood flow in real time throughout the B-mode image. The advantages of CCDS in the evaluation of the carotid arteries have been described in the previous chapter. This chapter will discuss the evaluation of normal vertebral arteries using CCDS and will describe findings associated with various pathological conditions as a basis for both diagnosis and basic clinical studies.

Examination technique

A color-coded Doppler sonography instrument equipped with both 7.5 and 5 MHz linear array transducers should be used. Patients are examined in the supine position with the shoulders as far caudad as possible and the head rotated slightly to the opposite side. At the beginning of the examination the probe is positioned over the lateral cervical region parallel to the carotid artery. The middle portion of the vertebral artery can then be identified by a slight lateral shift of the transducer associated with angulation as necessary to bring the transverse processes of the cervical spine into view; this scan plane will demonstrate the intertransverse portion of the vertebral artery which can then be traced caudad to the subclavian artery and cephalad to the base of the skull. For the visualization of the cranial portion of the vertebral artery ("atlas loop") the scanhead is positioned just below the mastoid process in an oblique plane pointing to the contralateral eye of the patient. The sensitivity of the system for the detection of motion is set individually for each patient to the point at which color "noise" is observed and is then reduced to just below the noise threshold. The color display is both directly evaluated and used as a guide for location of sampling sites for Doppler waveforms from all portions of the vertebral artery. Maximum and minimum velocities as well as resistive indices are measured. The resistive index (RI) is calculated from the equation $RI = 1 -$ (end-diastolic velocity / peak systolic velocity).

For purposes of analysis we subdivided the extracranial course of the vertebral artery into 3 segments: segment 1 includes the origin and proximal portion of the artery; segment 2 consists of the intertransverse portion; segment 3 covers the part where the artery encircles the lateral mass of the atlas ("atlas loop"). Proper visualization of the different segments of the vessel and adequate color display of blood flow are necessary. Special attention is paid to narrowing of the color-coded lumen with focal decrease in color saturation (indicating increased flow velocity) and the presence of a color mosaic pattern (representing turbulent flow). To determine whether flow reversal is present, vertebral artery flow direction is always compared with the ipsilateral common carotid artery.

If flow is not evident with conventional settings, "slow flow" sensitivity settings are then used in order to identify minimal blood flow. Detailed vascular wall analysis is performed using the expanded area of interest (magnification without loss of resolution) capability of the scanner in order to identify non-stenosing atheromatous lesions.

Normal vertebral arteries

Segment 2 of each vertebral artery (VA) can be identified by the characteristic intertransverse course of the vessel medial to the vertebral vein, and by hemodynamic characteristics (high diastolic flow) (Figs. 1, 2). The latter is also confirmed by spectral waveform analysis (Fig. 3). In many cases, the vertebral vein, or more commonly a vertebral venous plexus, can be seen descending parallel to the vertebral artery (Fig. 4). The vessel is then traced downward to the subclavian artery with demonstration of the origin and proximal portion of the artery (Figs. 5, 6). Following the course of the vessel up to the C1-2 level the atlas loop can be demonstrated as a curved vessel with a distinct change in color because of the

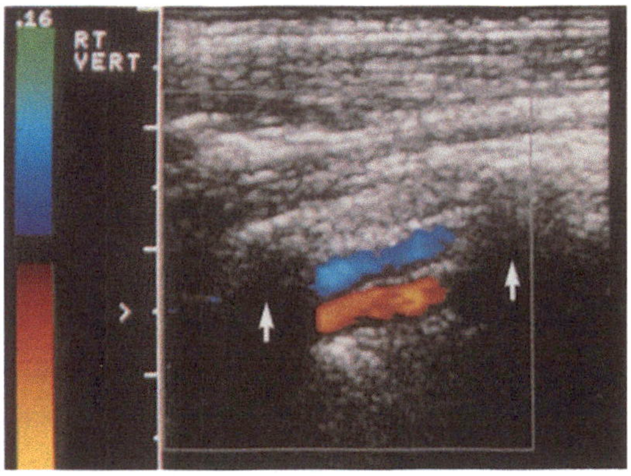

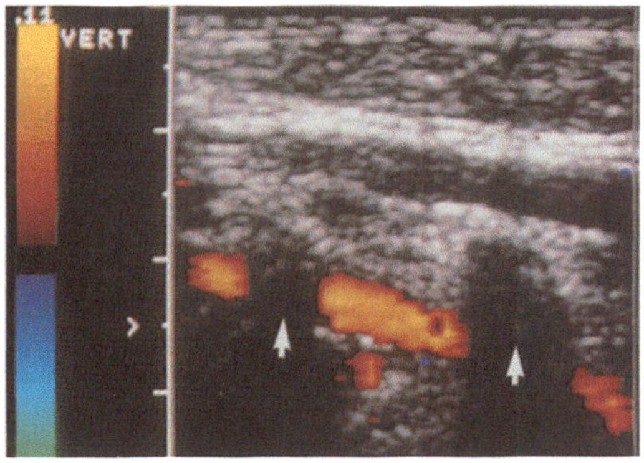

Fig. 1. (left) Color-coded Doppler sonogram of segment 2 of normal vertebral artery (red) and vertebral vein (blue); note shadowing from the transverse processes of the cervical spine (arrows)

Fig. 2. (right) Longitudinal CCDS image of segment 2 of a normal vertebral artery demonstrating gaps in the color image due to transverse process shadowing (arrows)

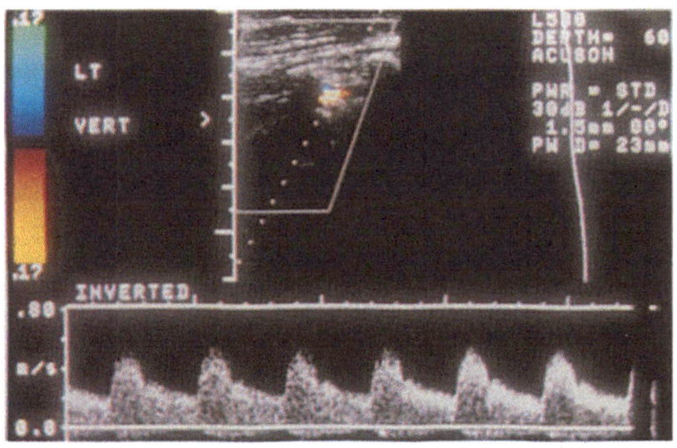

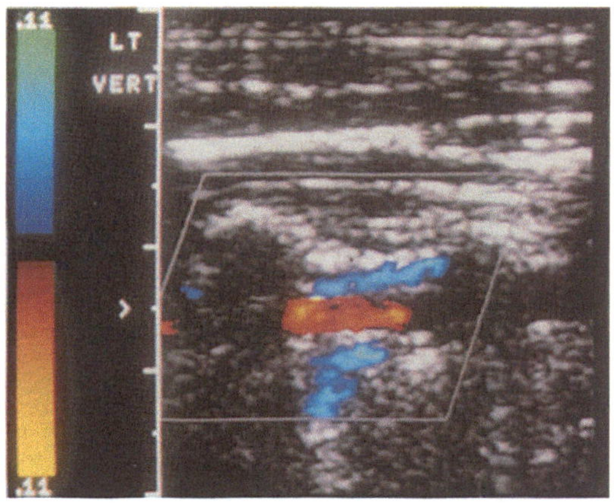

Fig. 3. (left) CCDS of segment 2 of vertebral artery in longitudinal view with spectral tracing illustrating high diastolic flow typical of a low-resistance vessel

Fig. 4. (right) Segment 2 of VA illustrating vertebral venous plexus (blue)

changing flow direction with respect to the transducer. Next to the atlas loop the surface of the posterior arch of the atlas is shown as a curvilinear echo with shadowing (Figs. 7, 8).

Considering the widespread use and the excellent results of duplex scanning for the detection of carotid artery disease it is surprising that only a few studies are devoted to duplex sonography of the vertebral arteries. Ackerstaff et al. reported that of 117 vertebral arteries studied, 31 could not be identified with the duplex scanning system. Moreover, the duplex scan did not satisfactorily display the origin of the vertebral artery in 28 vessels.

In contrast to Ackerstaff et al., Touboul et al. were able to visualize the pretransverse and intertransverse segments in all of 50 healthy subjects by duplex sonography. The vessel origin was identified in 94% of the cases on the right and in 60% on the left; they did not evaluate the upper segment of the vertebral artery. In our own study of 84 vertebral arteries of patients with no history or physical

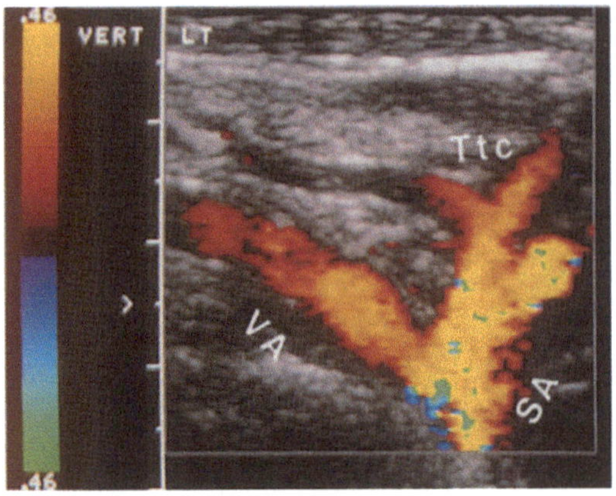

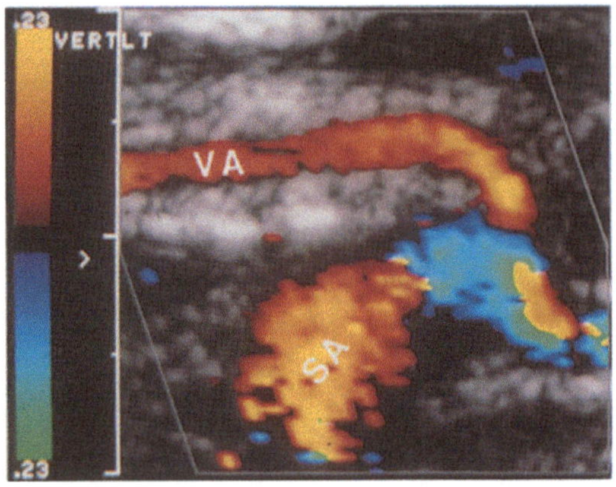

Fig. 5. (left) CCDS of segment 1 which includes a portion of the subclavian artery (SA) and the origin and proximal portion of a normal vertebral artery; the thyrocervical trunk (Ttc) is demonstrated superficial to the vertebral artery

Fig. 6. (right) CCDS of segment 1 with VA emerging from the subclavian artery and demonstration of a long segment of the proximal portion of the artery

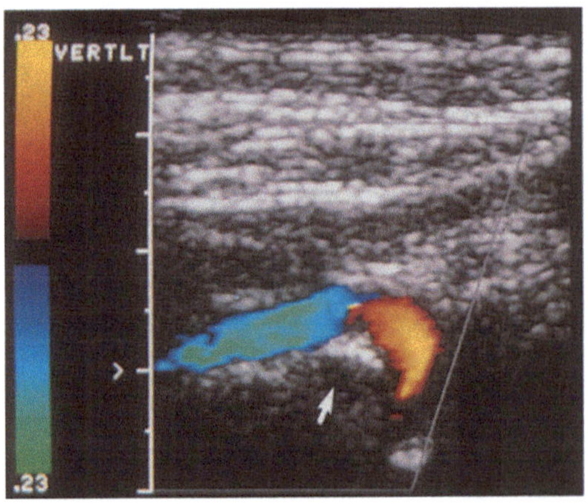

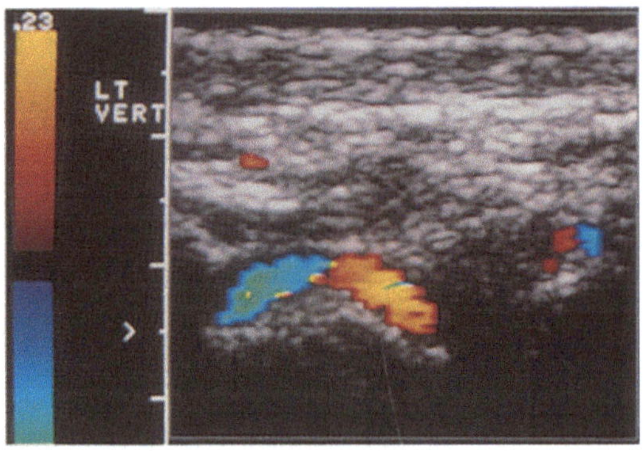

Fig. 7. (left) CCDS of segment 3 in an oblique plane showing normal vertebral artery (atlas loop) and posterior arch of atlas (arrow)

Fig. 8. (right) Another example of vertebral artery atlas loop with distinct change of color related to changing direction of flow relative to the transducer

signs of vertebrobasilar disease, segment 2 was visualized bilaterally in all patients. The atlas loop could be visualized in 76.2% (n=32) on the right and 85.7% (n=36) on the left side. In all patients the proximal segment was well seen except for the origin from the subclavian artery. The origin could be visualized in 88.1% (n=37) on the right and 66.7% (n=28) on the left. The peak systolic velocity ranged from 19 to 98 cm/sec (mean: 56 cm/sec), and the peak diastolic velocity from 6–30 cm/sec (mean: 17 cm/sec). The resistive indices ranged from 0.62 to 0.75 (mean: 0.69). The mean duration of the examination of both sides was about 15 minutes. Our results are similar to those of Touboul et al. with respect to the proximal and intertransverse portion of the vertebral artery, but we were also able to visualize the "atlas loop" of the vertebral artery in a high percentage of our patients. Our study demonstrates that CCDS allows identification and visualization of the three segments of the extracranial vertebral arteries in a high percentage of examinations, including the proximal segment with the vessel origin as well as the upper portion where the vertebral artery encircles the lateral mass of the atlas. The origin of the left vertebral artery from the subclavian artery is more difficult to visualize than the right one, perhaps because of the deeper course of the left subclavian artery as compared to the right side. It should also be noted that the left vertebral artery emerges directly from the aorta in 8% of individuals.

CCDS of the vertebral arteries may also be suboptimal in the presence of more posteriorly-oriented origins and in cases where there is marked tortuosity of segment 1. In obese patients with short necks it is difficult to position the transducer probe adequately for visualization of the "atlas loop" (segment 3) of the artery; in such cases, continuous wave Doppler may still be useful since it may be possible to obtain useful waveform information even if actual visualization is not possible.

Pathological findings

Hypoplastic arteries

The vertebral arteries are frequently asymmetric. The non-dominant artery is sometimes very small and does not participate in the formation of the basilar trunk. Until now there have been no accepted angiographic or sonographic criteria for hypoplastic vertebral artery (VA). In our study we have routinely made use of slow flow sensitivity settings when flow in the VA was not evident using conventional sensitivity values; this allows display of a thin string of color in hypoplastic arteries (Figs. 9, 10). This feature can be assessed in the intertransverse portion (segment 2) of the artery, but because of small vessel caliber identification of the vessel near its origin and in the atlas loop becomes impossible. In all cases spectral tracings are obtained to confirm the color-flow findings.

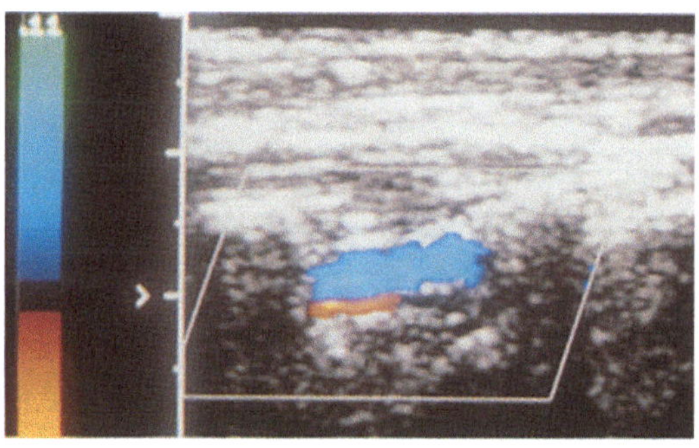

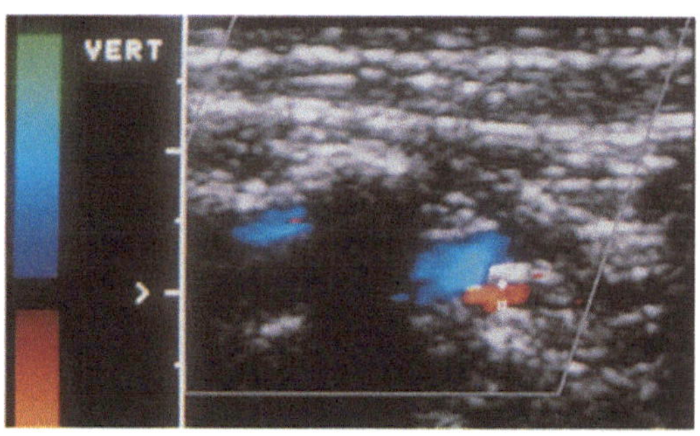

Fig. 9. (left) CCDS of hypoplastic VA visualized as a thin string of red color medial and parallel to a normal vertebral vein (blue)

Fig. 10. (right) Another example of VA hypoplasia with a string of red color adjacent to the descending vertebral vein (blue)

Stenosis

Frequency of atherosclerotic lesions has been found to be equivalent in the carotid and vertebrobasilar system from postmortem studies on selected patients with cerebrovascular disease. The most common site of stenosis or occlusion was at the VA origin from the subclavian artery. Fisher et al. described the lesion near the origin as stenosis with a ring-like configuration; more rarely, thickening of the posterior wall was found. High-grade stenoses are readily identified by CCDS because of visible reduction in diameter (facilitated by color-coding of the residual lumen) and direct visualization of hemodynamic abnormalities, particularly post-stenotic turbulence (Figs. 11, 12). Reports in the literature about the reliability of Doppler sonography in the diagnosis of stenotic lesions in the vertebral arteries are disappointing, with only 30% of all angiographically identified lesions being correctly diagnosed on the basis of the Doppler findings. In our study no false positive result of CCDS in comparison to angiography was recorded in the small (n = 5) group of patients with high-grade stenosis. High-resolution sonography is also able to detect atheromatous lesions of the proximal VA even in the absence of significant stenosis; the ability to analyze the surface and structural characteristics of the plaque (Figs. 13, 14) may be of some importance in identifying potential sources of local (artery to artery) embolism.

Occlusion

A diagnosis of a VA occlusion is possible if no color-coding of the artery can be identified in the readily accessible intertransverse segment even though the vessel walls can be seen on B-mode imaging. A further differentiation of occlusion from aplasia of the VA is possible when a proximal stump at the site of origin from the subclavian artery can be identified. It should also be noted that there may be reconstitution of a proximal occlusion, evidenced by patency of the atlas loop on

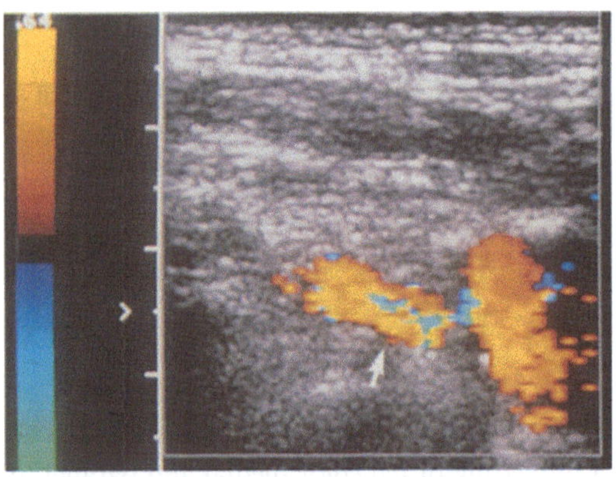

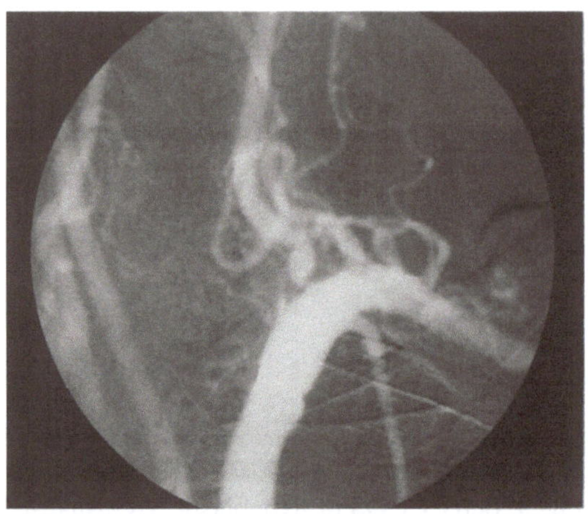

Fig. 11. (left) High-grade stenosis of VA origin with typical post-stenotic color mosaic indicating turbulent flow (arrow)

Fig. 12. (right) Aortic arch angiogram demonstrating a short segment high-grade VA origin stenosis

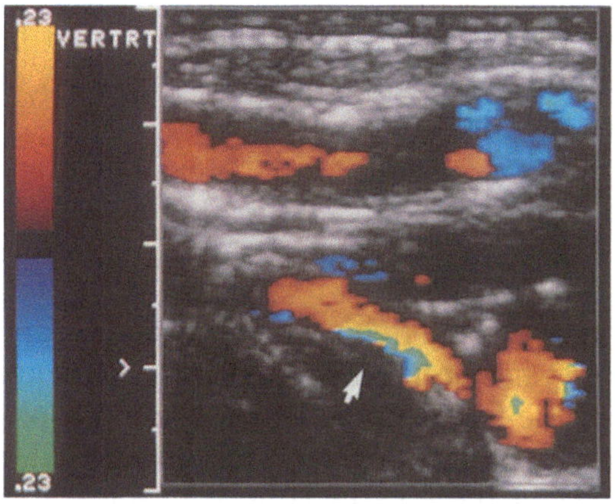

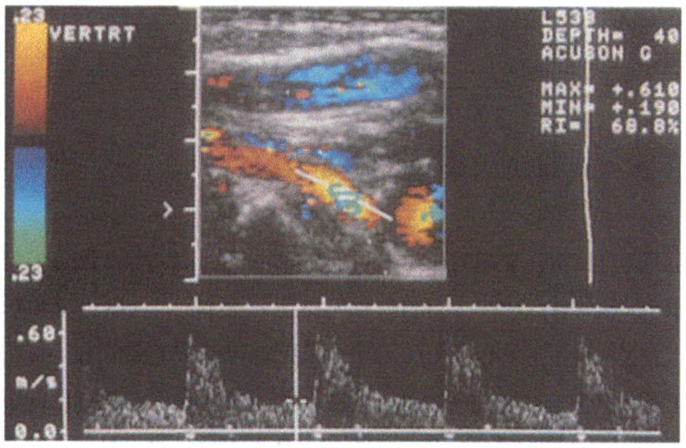

Fig. 13. (left) Proximal portion of VA in longitudinal color-coded Doppler sonogram; note atheromatous lesions of posterior wall without significant stenosis (arrow)

Fig. 14. (right) Spectral tracing from the same patient shows no significant velocity increase and no spectral broadening to suggest turbulent flow

CCDS (Figs. 15, 16); vessels which may contribute flow in such cases include the deep cervical artery, muscular branches of the thyrocervical trunk, the ascending pharyngeal artery, and the occipital artery branch of the external carotid artery.

Dissection

An advantage of identification of the atlas loop by CCDS is demonstrated in patients with dissection of the VA. This is a recently recognized pathological process which should be considered in the diagnosis of vertebro-basilar ischemia, especially in young people or when usual risk factors are lacking. The close relationship between the VA and the cervical spine explains why traumatic dissections are predominant. The third portion of the VA, especially in the C1-C2 interspace,

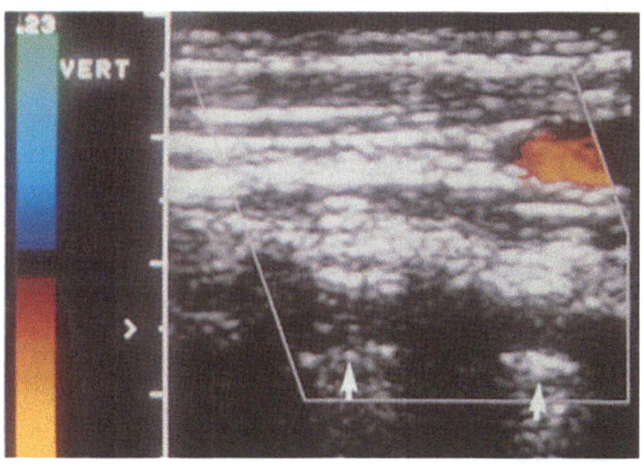

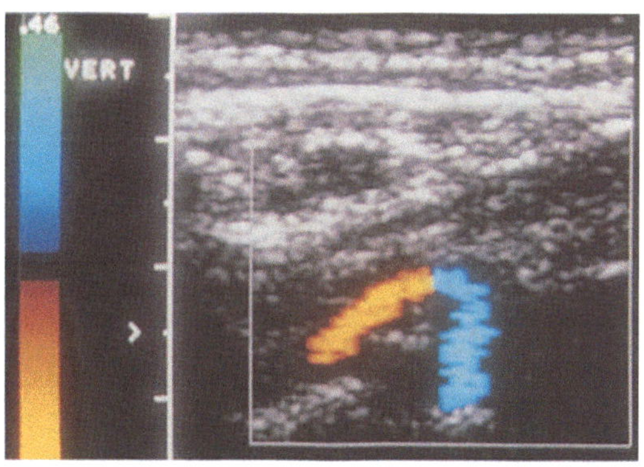

Fig. 15. (left) Occlusion of VA: absence of color flow in the intertransverse segment despite good demonstration of the vessel walls on the B-mode image (arrow)

Fig. 16. (right) Patency of the atlas loop confirmed by color-coding of segment 3; this patient had a proximal VA occlusion with reconstitution of the atlas loop from cervical collaterals

is the most common site of traumatic dissection. Regular or irregular narrowing of the VA (generally segmental) may be observed (Fig. 17). This finding should be considered strongly suggestive of vertebral artery dissection if there is a history of previous neck trauma and/or lack of other risk factors.

VA course abnormalities

Tortuosity and kinking are frequently observed in the first segment of the VA and more rarely in the second and third. Tortuosity has been shown to increase with age and may be due to atheromatous lesions of the fibrous type which cause atrophy of the media with resultant dilatation and elongation of the vessel. Using CCDS it is easy to follow the course of the vessel in these cases (Fig. 18). Sometimes kinking of the VA can be identified in the intertransverse portion of the vessel, although the distance between foramina in the transverse processes is short (Figs. 19, 20). Tortuosities rarely have hemodynamic consequences since they are not commonly associated with significant stenosis.

Cervical tumor with VA displacement

While any part of the cervical VA can be related to a tumor, the second and third portions are more likely to be involved since in these locations the VA is relatively

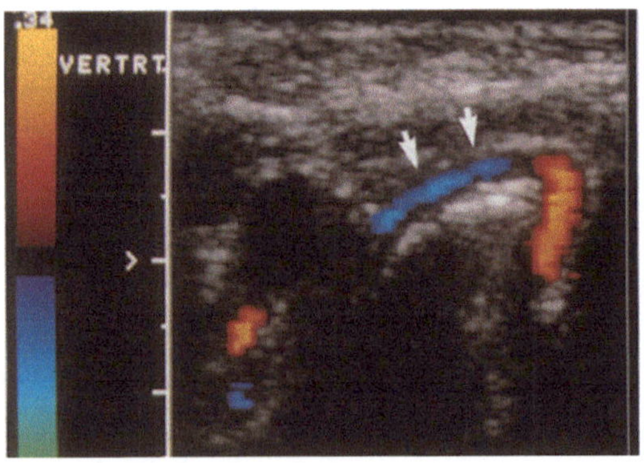

a

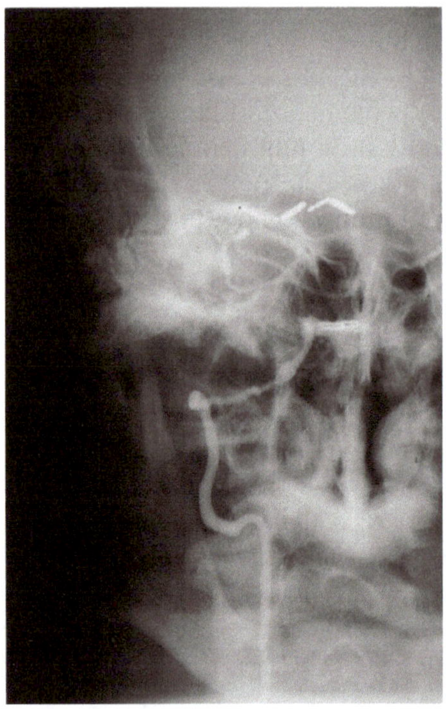

b

Fig. 17. Dissection of VA in the third portion (atlas loop) which is the most commonly involved site in cases of traumatic dissection. Segmented regular narrowing of VA is demonstrated in ***a***. (arrows) ***b***: Angiogram of same patient

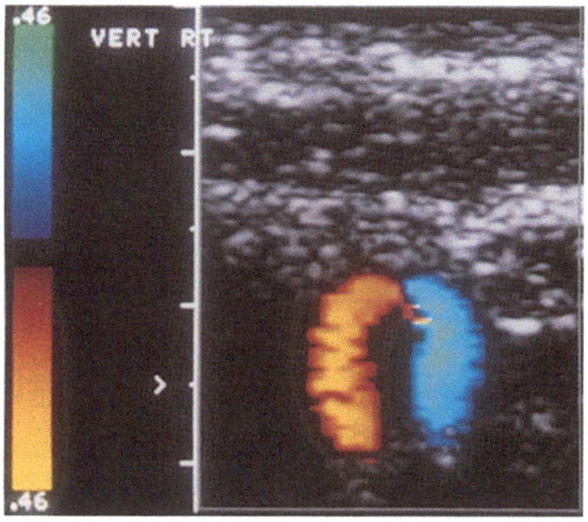

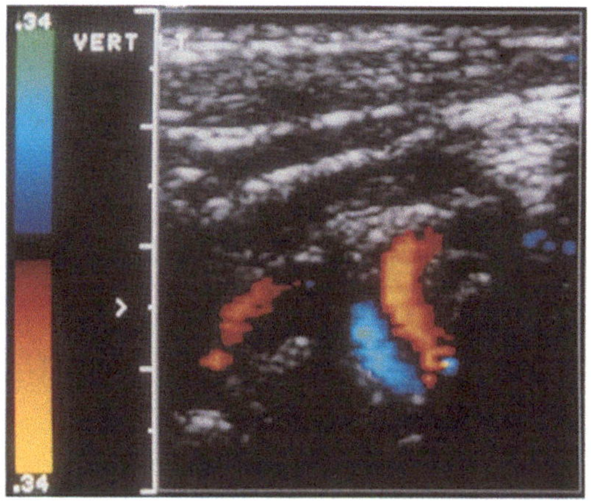

Fig. 18. (left) Tortuosity of segment 1 of the VA is readily apparent by CCDS in this case of 360° coiling of the vessel

Fig. 19. (right) Kinking of VA in segment 2 (intertransverse portion)

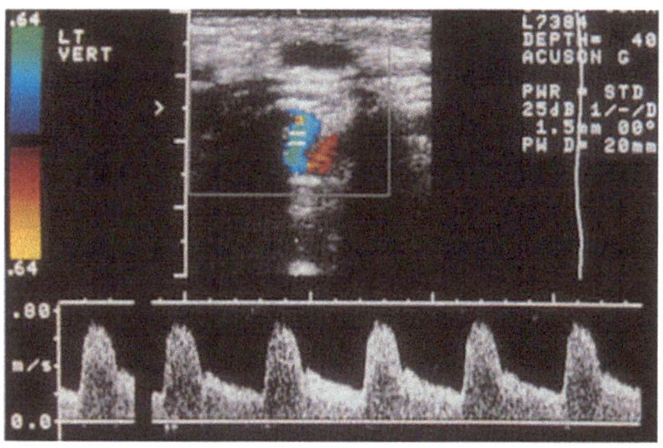

Fig. 20. Supplemental spectral tracing within the area of VA kinking in this example shows no waveform changes to suggest significant stenosis

fixed in position by the transverse process canal. CCDS is useful in the assessment of displacement and/or compression of the vessel lumen in these cases (Figs. 21, 22, 23).

Subclavian steal syndrome

When a subclavian artery stenosis or occlusion is proximal to the vertebral artery origin, flow from the contralateral vertebral artery can go to the basilar artery and then retrograde down the ipsilateral artery to reconstitute the subclavian artery distal to the area of abnormality. In marked contrast to the poor performance of continuous-wave Doppler ultrasound in the diagnosis of stenotic VA lesions, accuracy of diagnosis of subclavian steal syndrome has been reported to approach 100%. Color-coded images easily demonstrate flow reversal in the ipsilateral VA since color assignment will be opposite that in the common carotid artery and the

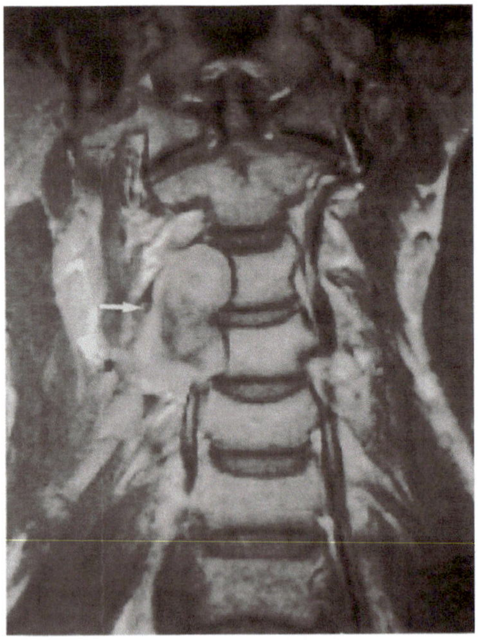

21

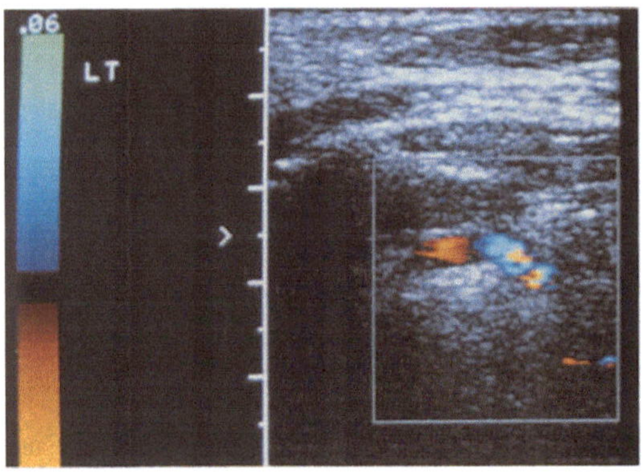

22

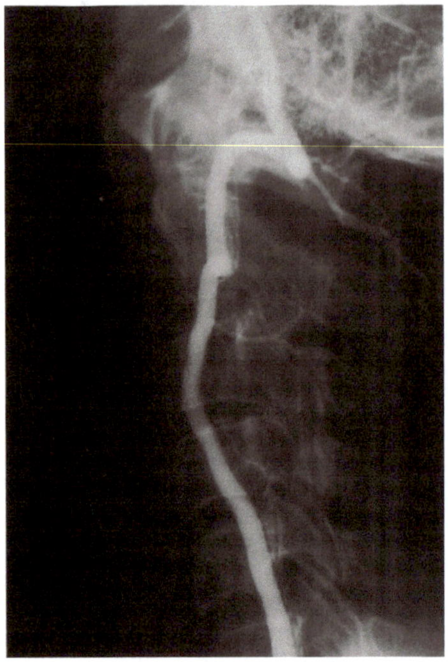

23

Fig. 21. MRI of cervical spine in the coronal plane shows recurrent neurofibroma at the level of C3-C4 on the right (arrow)

Fig. 22. CCDS of right VA in the longitudinal plane documents a ventral displacement by the tumor without significant stenosis

Fig. 23. (Same patient as Fig. 22) Selective right VA angiogram confirms the US diagnosis

same as that in neighboring vertebral veins (Figs. 24, 25). Since the reversed flow column is now supplying a high-resistance vascular bed (rather than the low-resistance intracerebral circulation) the spectral tracing will show decreased diastolic flow (Fig. 26).

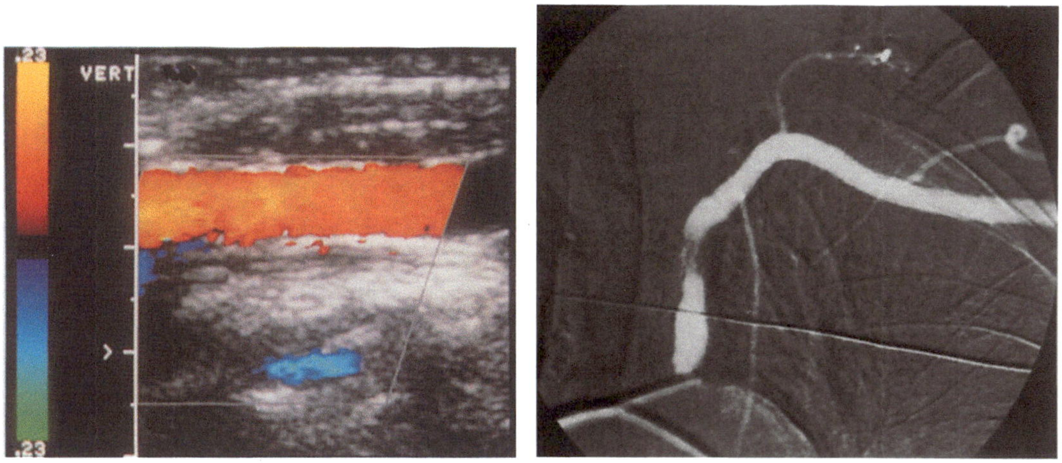

a b

Fig. 24. ***a*** Longitudinal view of common carotid artery (red) and VA (blue) on the same image indicating reversed VA flow in a patient with subclavian steal syndrome. ***b*** High grade stenosis of proximal subclavian artery on angiography

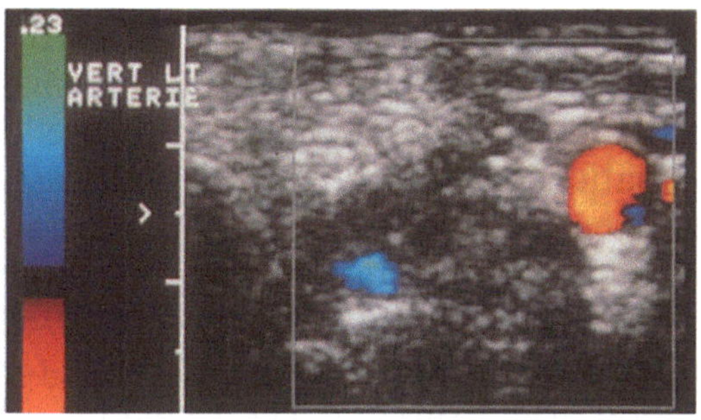

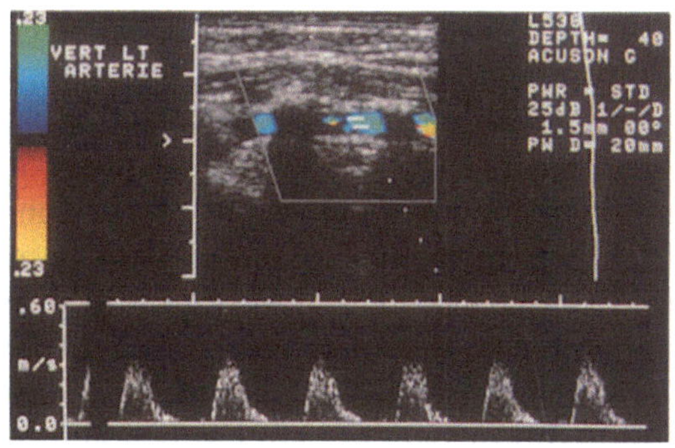

Fig. 25. (left) Transverse color-coded Doppler sonogram also shows reversed flow (blue) in VA compared to CCA (red)

Fig. 26. (right) Spectral tracing from a segment with reversed (blue) VA flow in a patient with subclavian steal syndrome demonstrates markedly decreased diastolic flow due to increased vascular resistance peripherally; Figs. 24–26 illustrate how CCDS facilitates the diagnosis of subclavian steal syndrome

Vertebral and subclavian surgery

CCDS is a useful technique for follow-up of patients following surgery of the subclavian and vertebral arteries. In patients who have undergone carotid-subclavian or vertebral-carotid bypass procedures CCDS is a noninvasive method of evaluation of direction of blood flow, lumen diameter, and hemodynamics in the ipsilateral vertebral artery (Figs. 27, 28).

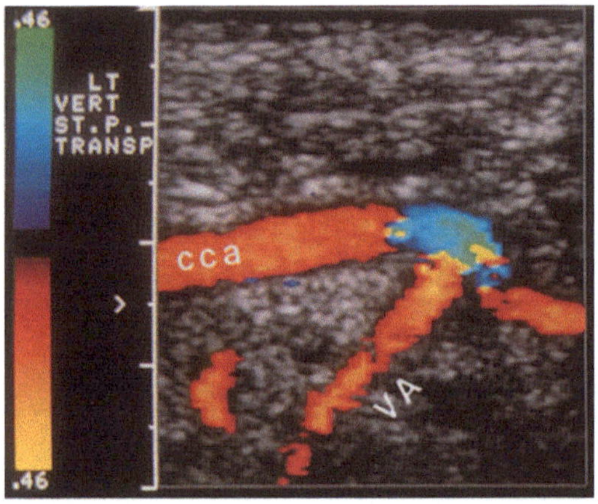

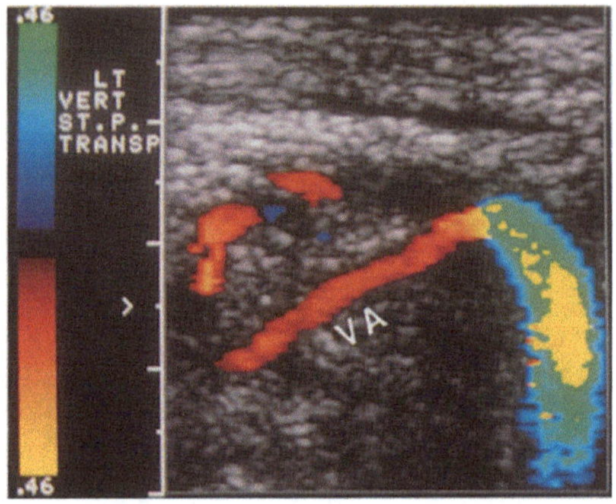

Fig. 27. (left) CCDS of a patient with reimplantation of VA to CCA shows the site of anastomosis as well as a longitudinal view of the proximal portion of VA

Fig. 28. (right) Longitudinal view of VA (red) with oblique view of CCA (blue) in a patient with VA reimplantation to the CCA

Conclusion

Color-coded Doppler sonography allows identification and visualization of the proximal, mid (intertransverse), and distal (atlas loop) portions of the extracranial vertebral artery in a high percentage of patients and has proved to be a useful noninvasive imaging technique for the evaluation of extracranial artery disease. CCDS is the method of choice for noninvasive evaluation of patients with generalized symptoms such as vertigo and dizziness and is useful in screening out those patients who may also need angiography, particularly if they are being considered for surgery. Conversely, angiography can often be avoided when CCDS is used for follow-up of patients after subclavian-vertebral artery surgery. The technique allows a comprehensive examination of the extracranial portion of all the vessels contributing to cerebral circulation, and since this can be accomplished in significantly less time than with previously available ultrasound techniques it becomes feasible to apply CCDS routinely in screening and follow-up protocols. Some limitations do exist; in cases where the vertebral origins are unusually deep (particularly if there is also vessel tortuosity) visualization of the origin may be marginal and stenotic areas could be missed. On the positive side, CCDS almost always allows adequate visualization of the mid-portion of the vertebral arteries as they course between the transverse processes, and the distal segment (atlas loop) of the vessels is also readily demonstrated in most cases. Other CCDS benefits include the ability to demonstrate such conditions as hypoplasia, tortuosity, dissection, subclavian steal syndrome and involvement of the vertebral artery by tumors of the cervical spine. On the whole, CCDS is presently the best noninvasive screening modality available for the patient with symptoms suggestive of abnormal vertebral artery function.

References

Ackerstaff RGA, Hoenefeld H, Slowikowski JM, Moll FI, Eikelboom BC, Ludwig JW (1984) Ultrasonic duplex scanning in atherosclerotic disease of the innominate, subclavian and vertebral arteries: A comparative study with angiography. Ultrasound Med Biol 10:409–418

Amaral JF, Grigoriev VE, Dorfman GS, Carney WI Jr (1989) Vertebral artery pseudoaneurysm. A rare complication of subclavian artery catheterization. Arch Surg 125:546–547

Bluth EI, Merritt CR, Sullivan M, Bernhardt S, Darnell B (1989) Usefulness of duplex ultrasound in evaluating vertebral arteries. J Ultrasound Med 8(5):229–235

Büdingen HJ, von Reutern GM, Freund JH (1982) Dopplersonographie der extrakraniellen Hirnarterien. Grundlagen, Methodik, Fehlermöglichkeiten, Ergebnisse. Thieme, Stuttgart New York

Clarisse J, Dobbelaere P, Francke JP, Julliot JP, Jomin M (1977) Superselective injection of the carotid and vertebrobasilar system using a coaxial catheter. J Neuroradiol 4:5–11

Davis PC, Nilsen B, Braun IF, Hoffman JC Jr (1986) A prospective comparison of duplex sonography versus angiography of the vertebral arteries. AJNR 7:1059–1064

Fisher CM (1961) A new vascular syndrome: "The subclavian steal syndrome". N Engl J Med 265:912–913

Fisher CM, Gore I, Obake N, White PD (1965) Atherosclerosis of the carotid and vertebral arteries extracranial and intracranial. J Neuropath Exp Neurol 24:455–476

Francke JP, Dimarino V, Pannier M, Argenson C, Libersa Cl (1980) Les arteres vertebrales. Segments atlantoaxoides V3 et intra-cranien V4 collaterales. Anatomia Clinica 2:229–242

Hutchinson EC, Yates PO (1957) Carotido-vertebral stenosis. Lancet I 2:2–8

Iraci G, Pardascher K, Fiore DL, Geros AM (1981) Vertebro-basilar transient ischemic attacks: An unusual clinical manifestation of a cervical aneurysmal bone cyst. Surg Neurol 16:251–255

Katirij MB, Reinmuth OM, Latachaw RE (1985) Stroke due to vertebral artery injury. Arch Neurol 42:242–248

Krayenbühl H, Yaşargil MG (1957) Die vaskulären Erkrankungen im Gebiet der Arteria vertebralis und Arteria basilaris. Thieme, Stuttgart

Krueger BR, Okazaki H (1980) Vertebrobasilar distribution. Infarction following chiropractic manipulation. Mayo Clin Proc 55:322–332

Louw JA, Mafoyane NA, Small B, Neser CP (1990) Occlusion of the vertebral artery in cervical spine dislocations. J Bone Joint Surg [Br] 72:679–681

Macke A, Macke-Ribert C (1978) L'artere carotide interne. Etude anatomique et microradiographique. Exploration endoluminale. These Med, Lille, pp 76

Nikitin IuM (1983) Ultrasound Dopplerography in the diagnosis of the subclavian steal syndrome. Zh Nevrpathol Psikhiatr 83:1295

Patel A, Toole JF (1965) Subclavian steal syndrome – reversal of cephalic blood flow. Medicine 44:289–303

Reutern GM von, Budingen HJ, Freund HJ (1976) Doppler-sonographische Diagnose von Stenosen und Verschlüssen der Vertebralarterien und des subclavian-steal-Syndroms. Arch Psychiatr Nervenkr 222:209

Reutern GM von, Pourcelot L (1978) Cardiac cycle dependent alternating flow in vertebral arteries with subclavian stenoses. Stroke 9:229

Ringelstein EB (1984) Ultraschalldiagnostik am vertebrobasilären Kreislauf. Ultraschall 5:215–223

Ringelstein EB, Kolmann HL, Kruse L (1984) Dopplersonographie der extrakraniellen Hirnarterien: In erster Linie ein didaktisches Problem. Ultraschall 4:182–187

Schwarz N, Buchinger W, Gaudernak T, Russe F, Zechner W (1991) Injuries to the cervical spine causing vertebral artery trauma: Case reports. J Trauma 31:127–133

Sherman DG, Hart RG, Easton JD (1981) Abrupt change in head position and cerebral infarction. Stroke 12:2–6

Touboul PJ, Bousser MG, Laplane D, Castaigne P (1986) Duplex scanning in normal vertebral arteries. Stroke 17:921–923

Touboul PJ, Mas JL, Bousser MG, Laplane D (1988) Duplex scanning in extracranial vertebral artery dissection. Stroke 19:116–121

Trattnig S, Hübsch P, Schuster H, Pölzleitner D (1990) Color Doppler Imaging of normal vertebral arteries. Stroke 8:1222–1225

Trattnig S, Schwaighofer B, Hübsch P, Schwarz M, Kainberger F (1991) Color-coded Doppler sonography of vertebral arteries. J Ultrasound Med 10:221–226

Vitek JJ (1989) Subclavian artery angioplasty and the origin of the vertebral artery. Radiology 170:407–409

White DN (1986) Vertebral sonography. In: Zwiebel WJ (ed) Introduction to vascular ultrasonography, 2nd edn. Grune & Stratton Inc, Orlando, pp 217–243

Wilkinson DL, Polak JF, Grassi CJ, Whittemore AD, O'Leary DH (1988) Pseudoaneurysm of the vertebral artery: appearance on color-flow Doppler sonography. Am J Roentgenol 151(5): 1051–1052

Yamaura A, Watanabe Y, Saeki N (1990) Dissecting aneurysms of the intracranial vertebral artery. J Neurosurg 72:183–188

5
CCDS evaluation of the arteries of the upper limbs

P. Hübsch and S. Trattnig

Introduction

In contrast to the clinical presentation of stenosis or occlusion in the carotid arteries or arteries of the lower limbs, arterial compromise in the upper extremities is often relatively asymptomatic and occurs less frequently. When symptoms are present they relate both to the location and severity of the lesion and to the degree of muscular exertion in the affected vascular bed. Figure 1 summarizes the major arteries of the upper extremity including their origins and their most important branches. Special attention should be given to the origin of the vertebral arteries from the subclavian arteries, and to the anatomic differences in the origins of the right and left subclavian arteries; it is these features which lead to the characteristic hemodynamic consequences of stenoses or occlusions of the brachiocephalic or subclavian arteries respectively, as will be discussed in more detail later in the chapter.

A thorough physical examination should be carried out before Doppler examination of any patient with suspected upper extremity arterial disease. Depending on the patient's history, this examination should include clinical tests like the Allen test for the detection of occlusion of the antebrachial or palmar arteries or the Adson test for the detection of a thoracic outlet syndrome; bilateral measurements of brachial blood pressure are mandatory.

Doppler examination can provide important information regarding the location and severity of arterial compromise. The etiology of the vascular abnormalities, however, cannot be determined on the basis of the Doppler findings alone since a variety of diseases (inflammatory changes of the arterial wall, post-traumatic lesions, arteriosclerosis) can lead to upper extremity ischemia and, in some cases, to associated conditions such as the subclavian steal syndrome.

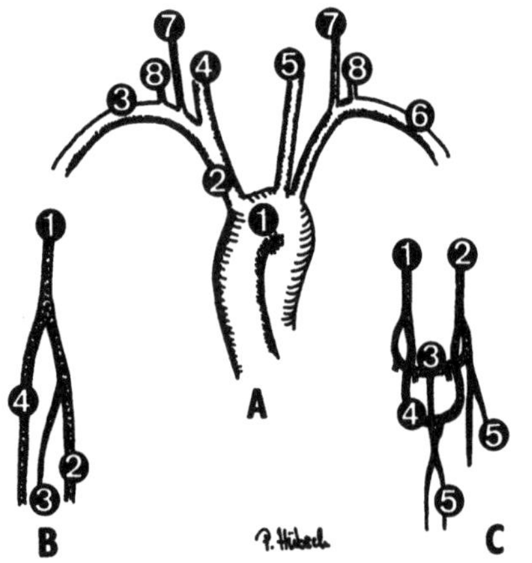

Fig. 1 a. Arteries of the thoracic outlet: (1) aortic arch (2) brachiocephalic artery (3) right subclavian artery (4) right common carotid artery (5) left common carotid artery (6) left subclavian artery (7) vertebral arteries (8) thyrocervical trunks

Fig. 1 b. Arteries of the arm: (1) brachial artery (2) ulnar artery (3) anterior interosseous artery (4) radial artery

Fig. 1 c. Arteries of the wrist and hand: (1) ulnar artery (2) radial artery (3) deep palmar arch (4) superficial palmar arch (5) digital arteries

Conventional duplex Doppler instruments are adequate for examination of the major arteries of the thoracic outlet and upper limb, but optimal evaluation of the small vessels of the hand and wrist, or assessment of arteriovenous malformations, requires color-coded Doppler capability. It is also true that CCDS facilitates rapid evaluation of flow status over a wide area, reducing examination time and enhancing diagnostic accuracy.

Examination technique

It is important that Doppler examination not be limited to a focal segment of the arterial system of the upper limb; all of the major vessels from the thoracic outlet to the wrist should be carefully examined. The origin of the brachiocephalic artery on the right and of the subclavian artery on the left cannot be directly visualized because of overlying bone. Limited assessment of these vessels can be obtained by using supraclavicular positioning of the scanhead near the sternoclavicular joint. By obtaining Doppler waveform information and measuring systolic and diastolic blood flow velocity on both sides using this approach it is possible to obtain important indirect information about the non-visualized portions of the vessels. Whenever arterial disease is suspected in the region of the thoracic outlet, the vertebral artery must also be evaluated to determine whether a subclavian steal syndrome is present (see below). If initial evaluation of the vertebral artery shows normal direction of blood flow it is important to repeat the study after hand exercise to see if increased arterial demand in the arm leads to reversal of vertebral artery flow direction on either side.

The examination is carried out with the patient lying on their back with the arms in supination parallel to the body; elevation of the arms is used only for examination of the axillary artery and the proximal part of the brachial artery. The arteries of the hand are examined only if specifically indicated by the clinical presentation. The deep and superficial palmar arch and the digital arteries can be examined with linear scanheads of at least 7.5 MHz; delineation of these vessels is highly dependent on the experience and skill of the sonographer as well as the anatomic pattern in any given patient (for example, the deep and superficial palmar arch vessels are subject to considerable variability).

Normal findings

All the arteries of the upper limb are characterized by a flow pattern typical of vessels with high peripheral resistance: the end-diastolic blood flow velocity is zero and there may even be reversal of flow in early diastole (Fig. 2).

As noted above, the origin of the subclavian artery on the left side is rendered inaccessible to direct visualization by interposed bony structures, as is the major part of the brachiocephalic artery (Fig. 3). It is still possible, however, to demonstrate the point at which the brachiocephalic artery divides to form the right common carotid and subclavian arteries by using a supraclavicular approach at the sternal end of the clavicle; rarely (in patients with elongation of the aortic arch) the origin of the brachiocephalic artery may be demonstrated (Fig. 4).

The origin of the vertebral artery and the thyrocervical trunk (see Fig. 7 in the vertebral artery chapter) is easily seen in most patients. The proximal portion of the subclavian artery on both sides is best visualized using a supraclavicular approach; a subclavicular scanhead position will be necessary for visualization of the distal part of each subclavian artery (Fig. 5). The axillary and brachial arteries are easily identified, as are the ulnar and radial arteries (Fig. 6); the interosseous artery is too small and too deeply positioned for routine evaluation, but the clinical importance of this vessel is usually minimal. Figures 7 and 8 illustrate the use of CCDS for demonstration of the palmar arches and digital arteries.

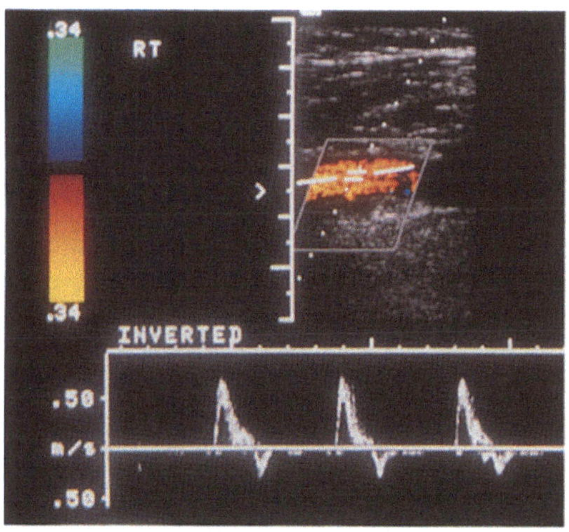

Fig. 2. Normal subclavian artery with Doppler waveform: there is a steep systolic velocity upstroke (short acceleration time) followed by a short interval with reversed blood flow; the end-diastolic blood flow velocity is zero

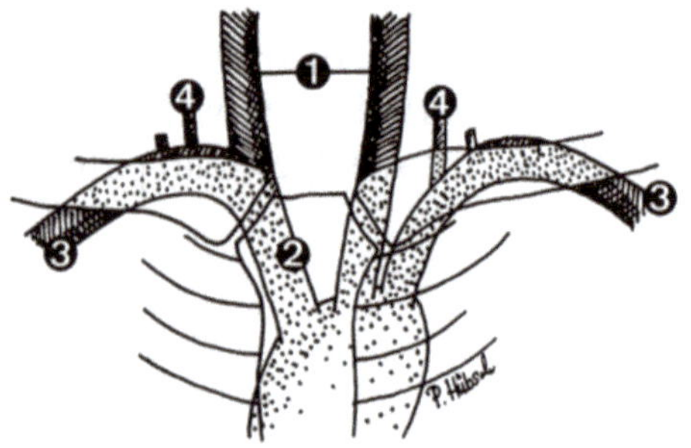

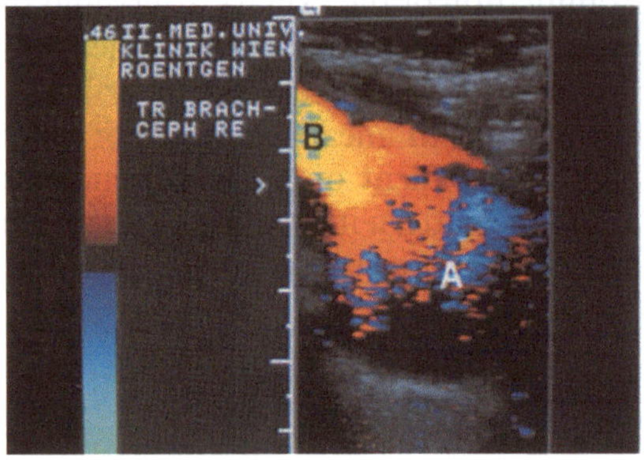

Fig. 3. (left) The main arteries of the thoracic outlet and their projection to the thoracic wall with respect to bony structures: the dotted parts of the vessels usually are not directly imaged sonographically (such as the origin of the brachiocephalic artery or the most proximal portion of the left subclavian artery). (1) common carotid arteries (2) brachiocephalic artery (3) subclavian arteries (4) vertebral arteries

Fig. 4. (right) Supraclavicular scanhead positioning usually shows the proximal part of the subclavian artery or the brachiocephalic artery. This approach may actually demonstrate the origin of the brachiocephalic artery (B) from the aorta (A) in asthenic patients with elongation of the aortic arch

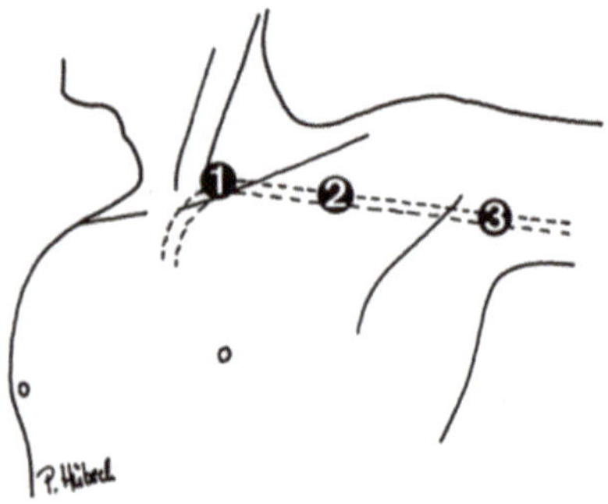

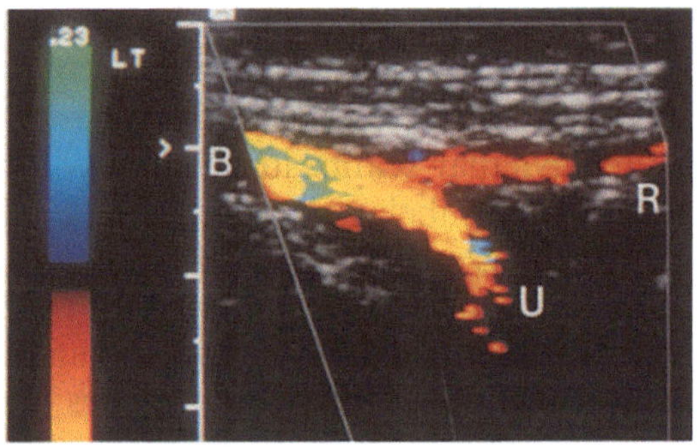

Fig. 5. (left) Optimal scanning approach to the subclavian and axillary artery: the proximal portion of the subclavian artery is best demonstrated by a supraclavicular probe position near the sternoclavicular joint (1); the more distal segments of the subclavian artery are best shown from an infraclavicular approach (2). For access to the axillary artery, the arm is elevated (3)

Fig. 6. (right) Branching of the brachial artery: CCDS clearly shows the origin of the radial (R) and ulnar (U) arteries from the brachial artery (B)

Pathological findings

Stenosis and occlusion

Stenoses or occlusions of the arteries of the upper limb are considered to be relatively rare in comparison with the incidence of such lesions in the lower extremities. It is quite possible that this impression is misleading due to the relative lack of symptoms when arterial compromise is present in the upper extremity, often confined to a feeling of fatigue in an arm after exercise; such limited symptomatol-

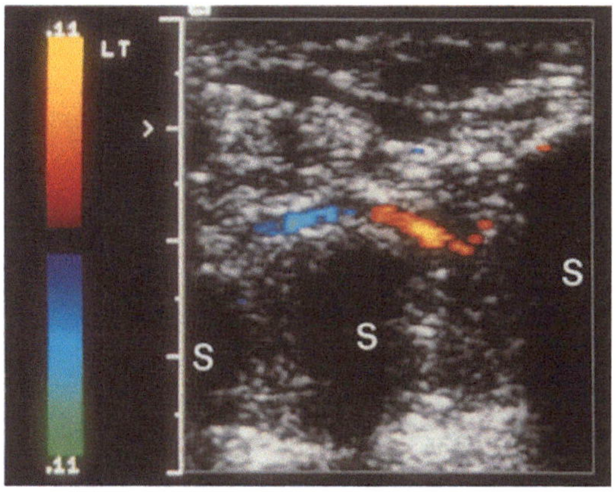

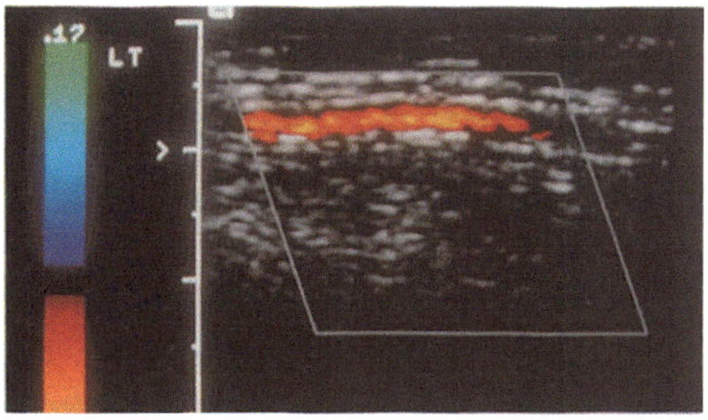

Fig. 7. (left) Deep palmar arch (transverse section at the level of the metacarpals): CCDS allows easy identification of the vascular structures (in contrast to the difficulty of vessel demonstration by gray scale ultrasound in this anatomic location). S = shadowing by metacarpal bones

Fig. 8. (right) Arteria princeps pollicis. Even small vessels like the digital arteries can be readily seen by CCDS

ogy may not lead the patient to consult a physician (in contrast to claudication in the lower extremities, which tends to be more disruptive of normal daily activities). The common practice of obtaining blood pressure readings from only one upper extremity also limits routine identification of some cases of subclavian artery stenosis: if bilateral brachial blood pressure values differ by more than 20–30 mmHg (2.6–4 kPa) then subclavian or brachiocephalic artery stenosis should be suspected on the side with lower pressure.

The most commonly encountered site of arterial stenosis affecting the upper extremity is the origin of the left subclavian artery from the aortic arch. As previously noted, this is a site not generally visualized directly during duplex Doppler or CCDS examination, so evidence of stenosis must be sought indirectly through resulting hemodynamic changes. Maximum systolic blood flow in the ipsilateral subclavian and axillary artery decreases in comparison to the contralateral vessels; the time required to reach peak systolic flow velocity is prolonged on the affected side. These changes can be appreciated in real time when CCDS is used for examination; measurement and documentation of the changes are facilitated by obtaining Doppler waveform tracings (Figs. 9, 10). In cases of severe stenosis (Fig. 11) or occlusion, the blood flow direction in the vertebral artery on the side of the stenosis may be reversed (Figs. 12, 13); this hemodynamic pattern is referred to as subclavian steal syndrome. When the effect of the stenosis is less pronounced, flow reversal may only be seen in the vertebral artery during systole, with some flow in the normal direction continuing in diastole giving a "pendulum motion" pattern. Exercise of the hand on the affected side (or inflation and then release of a blood pressure cuff) will usually convert this back-and-forth pattern to one of reversal throughout the cardiac cycle.

CCDS is also useful in long-term follow up of patients after dilatation (percutaneous transluminal angioplasty or "PTA") of subclavian artery stenosis (Figs. 14, 15).

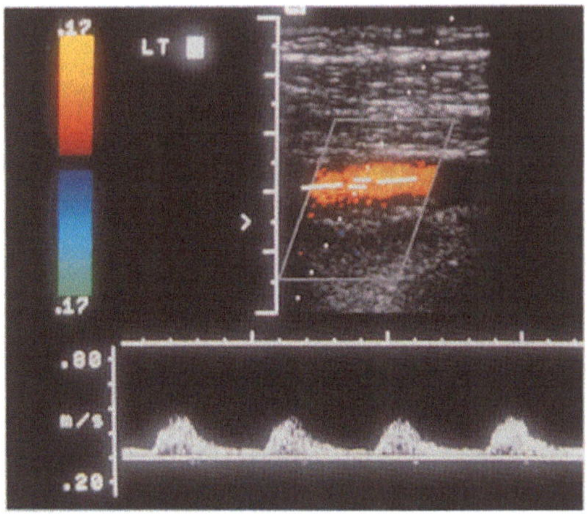

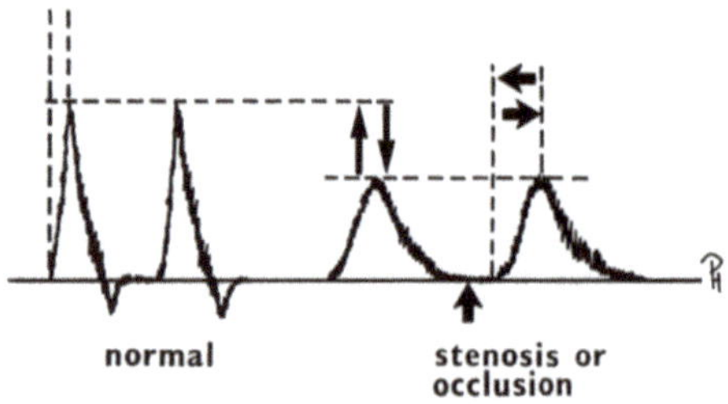

Fig. 9. (left) Pathologic alteration of blood flow in the left subclavian artery: the Doppler waveform suggests stenosis at the origin of the vessel (proximal to the transducer), which is not visible directly. Compare this waveform with the normal example in Fig. 2

Fig. 10. (right) Indirect signs of subclavian artery stenosis: The Doppler spectrum distal to an area of high-grade stenosis or occlusion shows reduced peak systolic velocity, prolonged acceleration time and loss of post-systolic flow reversal

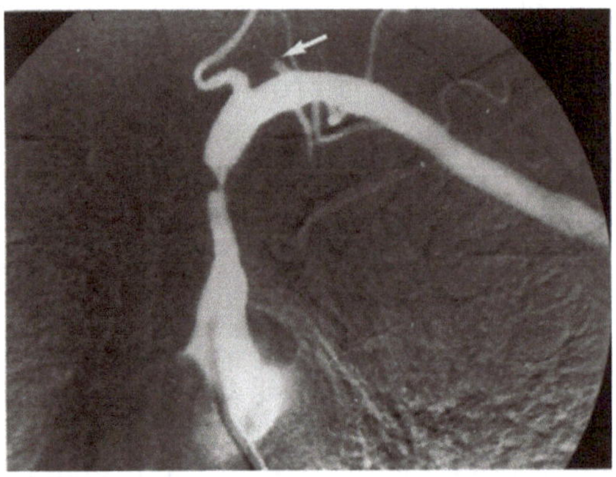

Fig. 11. Severe stenosis of the left subclavian artery shown by digital subtraction angiography. The vertebral artery (arrow) is not completely filled with contrast material. This does not indicate occlusion of the vessel; it is due to reversed flow in the vertebral artery (see Figs. 13, 14).

On the right side, stenosis is less common and may affect the subclavian artery as well as the brachiocephalic artery. When it is the brachiocephalic artery which is narrowed (Fig. 16) the carotid artery as well as the subclavian and vertebral arteries can be affected by the hemodynamic sequelae of the stenosis. Hemodynamic alterations of the vertebral artery usually precede changes in the carotid system; a majority of patients with brachiocephalic artery stenosis will have flow reversal in the ipsilateral vertebral artery, while a fully developed steal phenomenon with continuously reversed flow is rare in the carotid artery. More common findings in the carotid are alternating blood flow direction or simply a decrease in systolic blood flow velocity (Fig. 17).

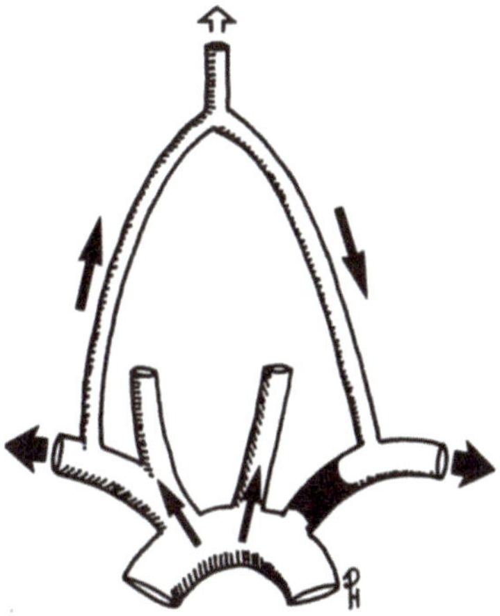

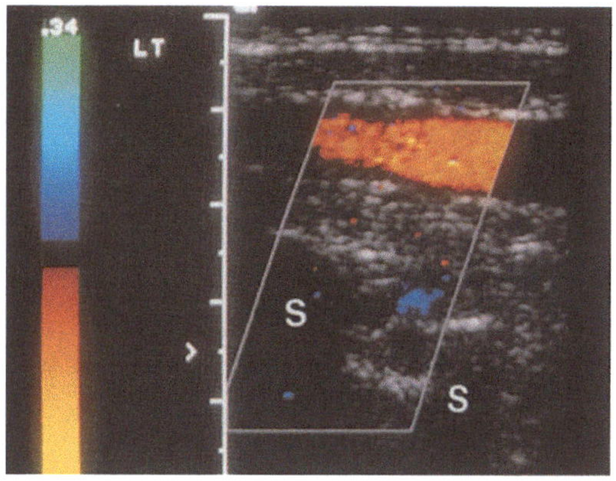

Fig. 12. (left) Summary of the hemodynamic consequences of left subclavian artery occlusion or high-grade stenosis: collateral blood suppy is provided by the vertebral artery system. This leads to flow reversal in the ipsilateral vertebral artery and may result in hypoperfusion of the basilar artery, leading to vertigo (especially during muscular exertion of the left arm)

Fig. 13. (right) Reversed flow direction in the left vertebral artery in the patient with subclavian artery stenosis shown in Fig. 11 ("subclavian steal"): the normally-directed blood flow in the common carotid artery is shown in red, whereas the vertebral artery is shown in blue (S = shadowing by transverse process of cervical vertebra). CCDS confirms patency of the vertebral artery as well as reversed flow direction

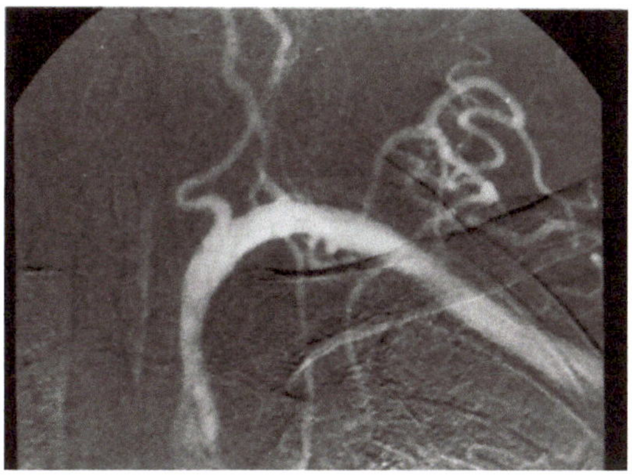

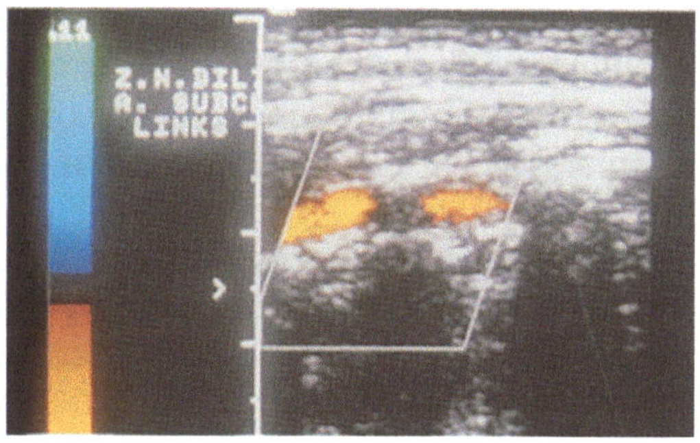

Fig. 14. (left) Angiogram of the left subclavian artery and its branches after angioplasty (same patient as in Fig. 11): the stenosis has been treated successfully by PTA. With restoration of normal flow direction in the vertebral artery there is now complete filling of the vessel lumen with contrast material

Fig. 15. (right) CCDS examination confirms normal direction of blood flow in the left vertebral artery following PTA of subclavian artery stenosis (same patient as in Figs. 11–14)

Pathologic changes of the subclavian artery *distal* to the origin of the vertebral artery, or changes at the level of the axillary artery, are most commonly associated with inflammation (Takayasu arteritis) or chronic trauma. The latter can be related to compression by a cervical rib or by muscle hypertrophy at the thoracic outlet, or to direct vessel damage due to unusual patterns of exertion as can occur with baseball pitchers and other athletes. Abduction and external rotation of the arm can cause compression of the axillary artery by the humeral head which can in turn

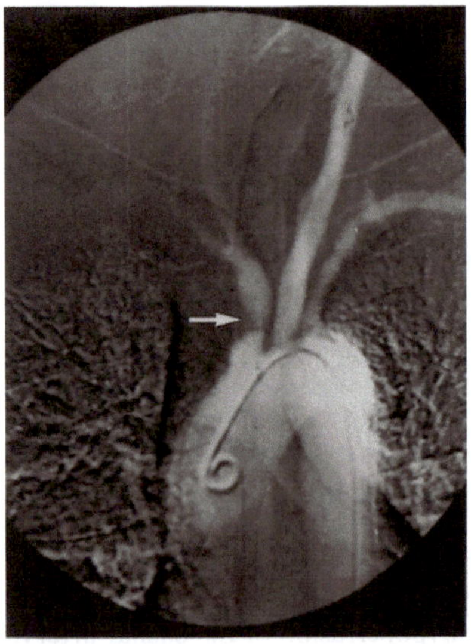

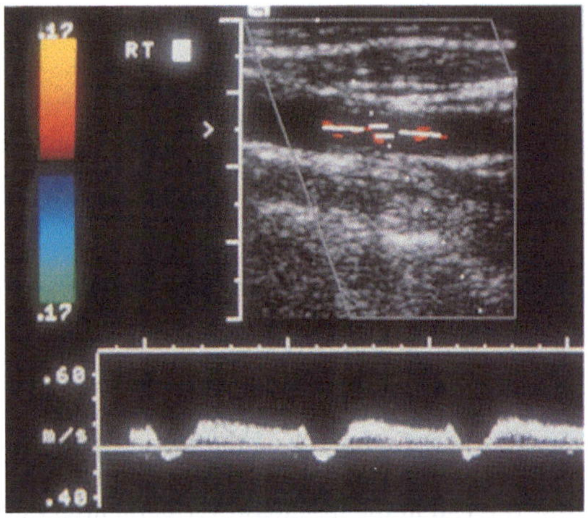

Fig. 16. (left) Severe stenosis of the brachiocephalic artery with poststenotic dilatation shown by digital subtraction angiography: the stenosis (arrow) leads to delayed delineation of right carotid and subclavian artery

Fig. 17. (right) Same patient as in Fig. 16: abnormal blood flow in the right common carotid artery with diminished velocity and absence of systolic velocity peaks. There is a periodic reversal of blood flow direction. Note the faint color display of the carotid artery due to slow blood flow

lead to chronic vascular trauma in persons involved in sports requiring repeated throwing motions. Chronic vascular trauma (one example is long-term occupational vibration trauma as encountered in operators of heavy machinery or pneumatic hammers) can also lead to stenosis or occlusion of the arteries of the forearm, wrist and hand.

The criteria for arterial stenosis or occlusion in the upper limb are in general similar to those used for the cerebral vessels with one important exception: since normal diastolic velocity values fall to (or below) zero, diastolic blood flow velocity cannot be used as an indirect indicator for distal occlusion. One exception to this rule is in patients with dialysis fistulas (see related chapter); another exception is when the cerebral arteries themselves are being evaluated for changes related to upper limb ischemia.

Vascular malformations

Vascular malformations can be divided into benign and malignant lesions. The very heterogeneous group of benign vascular malformations is perhaps best approached by considering three subgroups: the arteriovenous fistula, the arteriovenous malformation, and the hemangioma.

1. Arteriovenous fistulas

An A-V fistula is defined as a single *acquired* communication between an artery and a vein (with no intervening capillary bed); the cause is most commonly injury or vascular erosion. Clinical evaluation will reveal a thrill to palpation and a typical bruit on auscultation. The patient will experience problems in proportion to the size (shunt volume) and location of the fistula. The diagnosis is easily established with CCDS, with an appearance very similar to a dialysis fistula. The exact location of the shunt can usually be determined; a typical signal with high diastolic blood flow velocity will be present (Figs. 18, 19).

2. Arteriovenous malformations

In contrast to simple A-V fistulas, arteriovenous malformations (AVM's) are congenital lesions (hamartomas) with tumor-like properties. CCDS of an AVM will reveal multiple tortuous vessels (Fig. 20) with nearly continuous color display of

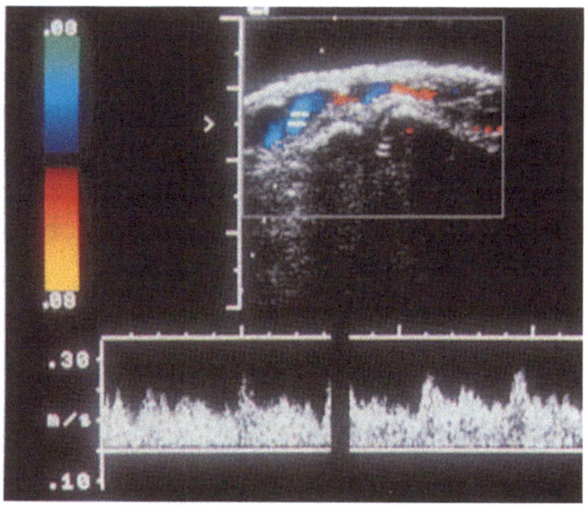

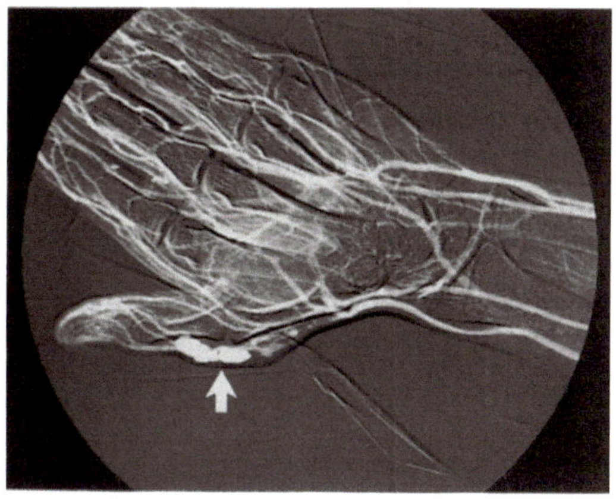

Fig. 18. (left) Arteriovenous fistula at the thenar level secondary to a dog bite: the shunt vessel is clearly delineated by color during systole and diastole. The Doppler waveform tracing shows high diastolic blood flow velocity typical of an arteriovenous shunt

Fig. 19. (right) Same patient as in Fig. 18: the diagnosis is confirmed by digital subtraction angiography of the hand. The shunt vessel is pointed out by an arrow

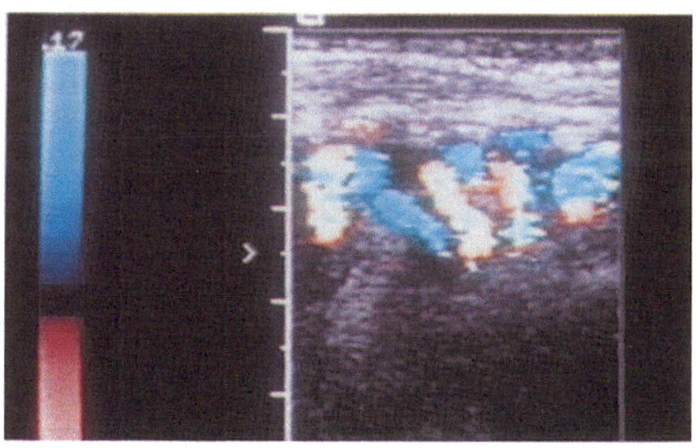

Fig. 20. Arteriovenous malformation presenting as an aggregate of coiled vessels

blood flow throughout diastole secondary to low resistance from multiple arterial-to-venous shunts. The Doppler waveform pattern will closely resemble that from an A-V fistula, but a single site of communication from the arterial to venous systems cannot be shown. The maximum blood flow velocity within the lesions can be very high (sometimes more than 1.5 m/s); as in other conditions resulting in such high flow velocities, perivascular color artifacts arising from tissue vibrations may be encountered (see Dialysis Fistula chapter for a detailed discussion of color-mosaic artifacts related to perivascular vibration).

With CCDS it is possible to delineate even small vessels and to prove the presence of A-V shunts even in such locations as the fingertip (Figs. 21, 22). Although the relationship to surrounding anatomical structures as well as the extent and nature of the lesions can be readily determined by CCDS, angiography is still necessary preoperatively to provide the surgeon with an overview of feeding arteries and draining veins.

3. Hemangiomas

Hemangiomas are also considered to be congenital. In contrast to A-V malformations, however, in most instances they do not contain arterial-to-venous shunts (an exception is in hemangiomas associated with the F.P. Weber syndrome – see below). Angiography may demonstrate a tumor "blush", but large feeding arteries or major draining veins are not present. CCDS signs of hypervascularity are usually absent in *capillary* hemangiomas because the blood flow in the capillary vessels is too slow for detection. Larger arteries within the lesion are characterized by a high-resistance blood flow pattern.

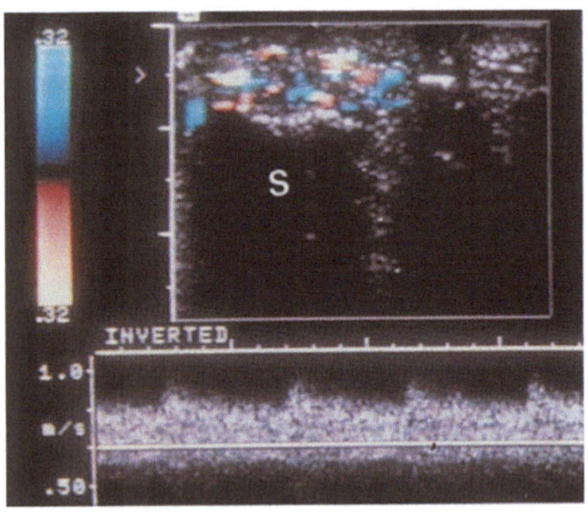

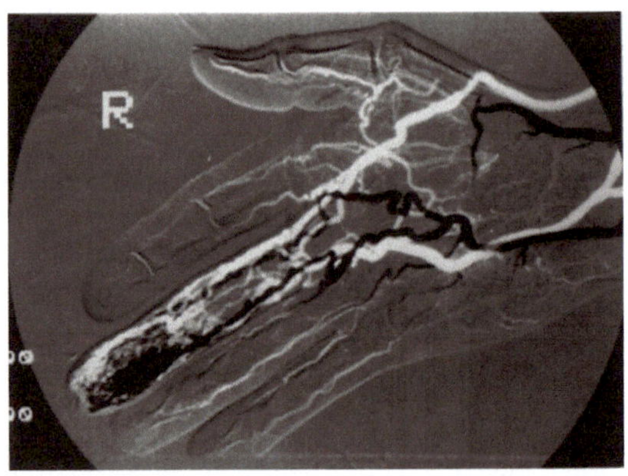

Fig. 21. (left) Arteriovenous malformation on a finger: CCDS reveals thickening of the soft tissue, which shows a rich bed of vascularity with evidence of arteriovenous shunts. (S: shadowing by phalangeal bone)

Fig. 22. (right) Digital subtraction angiography confirms the findings shown in Fig. 21: there is an arteriovenous malformation at the distal phalanx of the middle finger of the right hand; early venous return is clearly visible

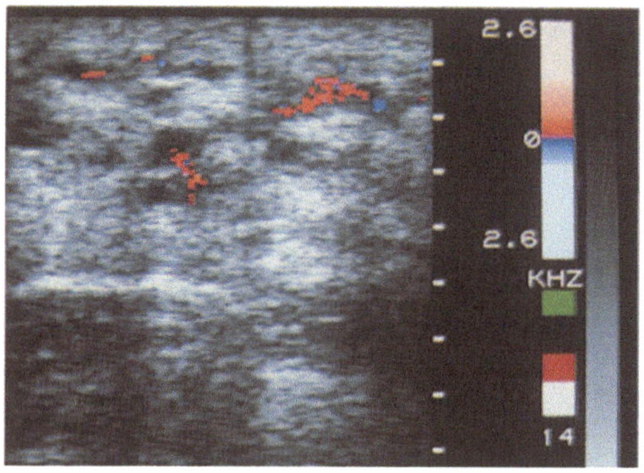

Fig. 23. Cavernous hemangioma with thickening of the soft tissue and sinusoid spaces containing blood. Because of very slow blood flow, color display can be obtained only by intermittent compression of the lesion with the scanhead ("sonopalpation")

Cavernous hemangiomas consist of large vessels which communicate to form a sponge-like lesion. While blood flow is also often slow in this type of hemangioma it is often possible to generate color flow patterns from within the lesion by applying intermittent pressure ("sonopalpation") with the scanhead (Fig. 23).

In certain clinical syndromes associated with hemangiomatous lesions it is important (with regard to therapy and prognosis) to detect A-V shunts. One example is the use of CCDS to differentiate the Klippel-Trenaunay syndrome (which is *not* associated with A-V shunts) from the F.P. Weber syndrome (which *is* characterized by A-V shunts).

4. Tumors

The demonstration by CCDS of a low echodensity mass without hypervascularity in association with a vascular lesion raises the possibility of a solid soft-tissue tumor, possibly of vascular origin, as with a hemangiopericytoma or an angiosarcoma (Fig. 24). Such a lesion may be indistinguishable from a hemangioma or A-V

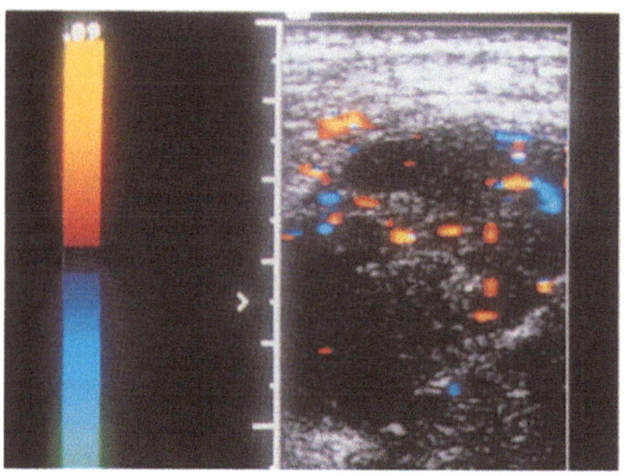

Fig. 24. Partially hypervascular hypoechogenic soft tissue mass found to represent a malignant hemangiopericytoma on histologic examination

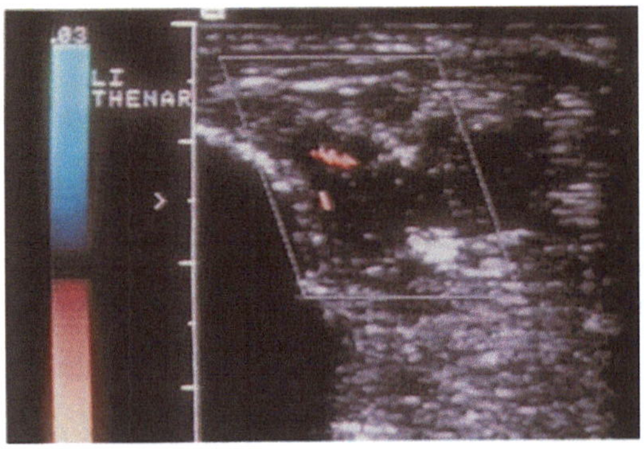

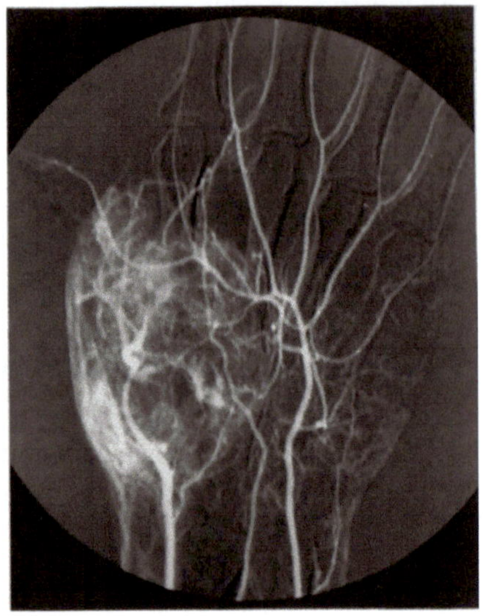

Fig. 25. (left) Hypoechogenic structures at the thenar level with some slightly hypervascular areas: surgically confirmed thrombosis in an arteriovenous malformation

Fig. 26. (right) Same patient as in Fig. 25: digital subtraction angiography shows inhomogeneous hyperperfusion of the lesion, but no early venous return

malformation by angiography, so the additional information from sonography may be important in narrowing the diagnostic possibilities. Even with the information from CCDS the findings are not pathognomonic since a vascular malformation with thrombosis can also have this type of appearance (Figs. 25, 26).

A-V malformations may be accompanied by skin abnormalities resembling those of Kaposi's sarcoma ("pseudo-Kaposi's sarcoma"). At the site of the vascular lesions, reddish-purple nodules and plaques may be observed. Even on histopathological examination there may be striking similarities between A-V malformations and Kaposi's sarcoma. Since the treatment of the two entities is very different (for example, radiation therapy is indicated in Kaposi's sarcoma but may actually be contraindicated in A-V malformations) it is important that the two conditions be accurately differentiated. CCDS may prove useful in this context because of its sensitivity in the detection of A-V shunts.

References

Baxter BT, Blackburn D, Payne K, Pearce WH, Yao JS (1990) Noninvasive evaluation of the upper extremity. Surg Clin North Am 70:87–97

Brunhoelzl C, von Reutern GM (1989) Hemodynamic effects of innominate artery occlusive disease. Evaluation by Doppler ultrasound. Ultrasound Med Biol 15:201–204

Earhart RN, Aeling JA, Nuss DD, Mellette JR (1974) Pseudo-Kaposi sarcoma. Arch Dermatol 110:907–910

Erickson SJ, Mewissen MW, Foley WD, Lawson TL, Middleton WD, Lipchik EO, Quiroz FA, Macrander SJ (1989) Color Doppler evaluation of arterial stenoses and occlusions involving the neck and thoracic inlet. Radiographics 9:389–406

Falk RL, Smith DF (1987) Thrombosis of upper extremity thoracic inlet veins: diagnosis with duplex Doppler sonography. AJR 149:677–682

Handl-Zeller L, Hübsch P, Hohenberg G, Schratter A, Wickenhauser J (1989) B-Bild und farbkodierte Dopplersonographie zur Bestrahlungsplanung bei Klippel-Trenaunay-Syndrom mit Kasabach-Merritt-Symptomatik. Ultraschall Med 10:41–43
Hübsch P, Trattnig S, Kainberger FM, Barton P, Karnel F (1991) Darstellung peripherer arteriovenöser Malformationen mittels FarbDoppler. Ultraschall Med 12:87–90
Lindenauer SM (1955) The Klippel-Trenaunay syndrome: Varicosity, hypertrophy and hemangioma with no arteriovenous fistula. Ann Surg 162:303–314
Lo CM, Yeung HY, Siu KF (1987) Misdiagnosed localized arteriovenous malformation. J Vasc Surg 6:419–421
Marshall E, Hatfield ST, Hatfield DR (1985) Arteriovenous malformation simulating Kaposi's sarcoma. Arch Dermatol 121:99–101
McCarthy WJ, Yao JS, Schafer MF, Nuber F, Flinn WR, Blackburn D, Suker JR (1989) Upper extremity arterial injury in athletes. J Vasc Surg 9:317–327
Reading CC, Charboneau JW, Allison JW, Cooperberg PL (1990) Color and spectral Doppler mirror-image artifact of the subclavian artery. Radiology 174(1):41–42
Reed AJ, Fincher RM, Nichols FT (1989) Takayasu arteritis in a middle-aged Caucasian woman: Clinical course correlated with duplex ultrasound and angiography. Am J Med Sci 298:324–327
Rohrer MJ, Cardullo PA, Pappas AM, Philips DA, Wheeler HB (1990) Axillary artery compression and thrombosis in throwing athletes. J Vasc Surg 11:761–768
Schulte M (1982) Arterielle Durchblutungsstörungen. In: Gross R, Schölmerich P (Hrsg) Lehrbuch der Inneren Medizin. Schattauer, Stuttgart New York
Trout HH, McAllister HA Jr, Giordano JM, Rich NM (1985) Vascular malformations. Surgery 97:36–41
Walker DW, Acker JD, Cole CA (1982) Subclavian steal syndrome detected with duplex pulsed Doppler sonography. Am J Neuroradiology 3:615–618

6
Color-coded Doppler sonography of the thyroid and parathyroid glands

P. Hübsch, F. Frühwald, and S. Trattnig

Introduction

Due to the superficial location of the thyroid gland and because of the high incidence of pathologic changes affecting this organ, it is an ideal structure for evaluation by ultrasound and especially color-coded Doppler ultrasound (CCDS). Transducers with frequencies of 5, 7.5, or even 10 MHz can be used depending on the depth of the particular region of interest. The use of such high frequencies allows extremely fine resolution of even small anatomic or pathologic structures within the thyroid and parathyroid glands as well as elsewhere in the neck.

Despite this degree of structural definition most of the intrathyroidal vessels are too small to be clearly demonstrated with B-mode ultrasound techniques. This has been a limiting factor in the application of duplex Doppler techniques to thyroid abnormalities. CCDS overcomes this limitation to some degree by providing flow information even for vessels too small to visualize on the B-scan image. The benefits and practical applications of this capability as related to differential diagnosis of pathologic changes in the thyroid and parathyroid glands will be outlined in this chapter. Two points must be emphasized: the first is that diagnosis must not rely solely upon the CCDS findings but must also carefully consider the gray scale B-scan characteristics of any mass; the second point is that CCDS as applied to thyroid and parathyroid evaluation is still a new technique subject to some controversy with respect to its role in the diagnosis of such conditions as malignancy. We will attempt to provide the most up-to-date information available regarding both the capabilities and limitations of CCDS.

Normal findings

The largest of the vessels feeding and draining the thyroid gland (Fig. 1 a, b) can usually be identified even by conventional gray scale B-mode ultrasound, but CCDS greatly facilitates their evaluation. The superior thyroid artery is the first branch arising from the external carotid artery; it courses from above the carotid bifurcation in a caudad direction to reach to upper pole of the thyroid lobe on each side. In most cases this vessel is quite easy to trace and actually serves as a marker for differentiation of the external from the internal carotid artery in cases where stenosing plaque or thrombus may lead to hemodynamic changes which obscure the usual waveform pattern differences used to distinguish the ECA from the ICA.

The inferior thyroid artery arises from the thyrocervical trunk. It is important to be aware that this vessel runs parallel to the vertebral artery at the level of the thyroid gland; caution must be exercised when evaluating possible vertebral artery compromise so that this vessel is not incorrectly identified as the vertebral artery.

The thyroid veins drain blood from the thyroid gland into the internal jugular vein and left brachiocephalic vein. Anastomotic venous connections between the superior and inferior thyroid veins are present at the surface of the gland (Fig. 2); these anastomoses can provide a collateral pathway for blood when there is thrombosis of the inferior portion of the internal jugular vein (as discussed in the chapter on veins of the upper extremity and neck). At the upper and lower poles of both thyroid lobes it is normal to find a large number of vessels representing branches of the superior and inferior thyroid arteries and veins (Fig. 3). It is important to become comfortable with this pattern in normal subjects to avoid misdiagnosis of a pathologic vascular lesion or hypervascular nodule.

The appearance of the thyroid gland in gray scale B-mode ultrasound images is well documented: a very characteristic finely homogeneous echotexture. This

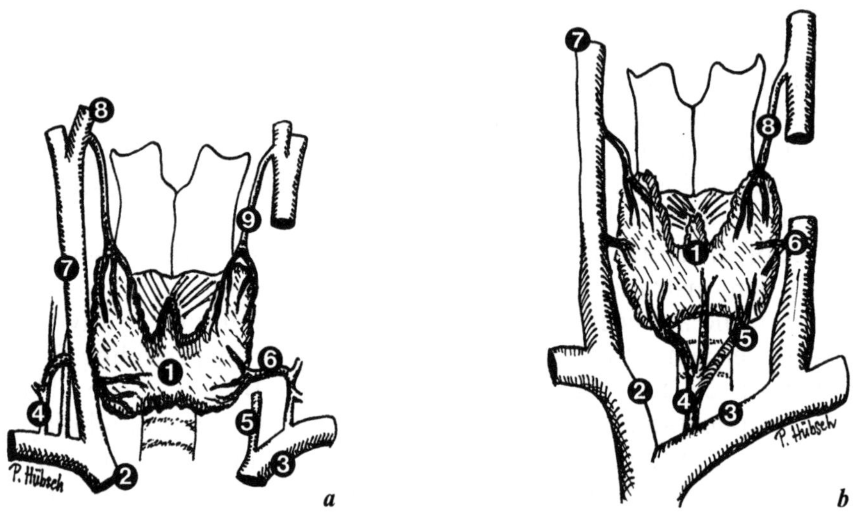

Fig. 1 a. Arteries of the cervical region and of the thyroid gland: (1) thyroid gland (2) brachiocephalic artery (3) left subclavian artery (4) thyrocervical trunk (5) vertebral artery (6) inferior thyroid artery (7) common carotid artery (8) external carotid artery (9) superior thyroid artery

Fig. 1 b. Veins of the cervical region and of the thyroid gland: (1) thyroid gland (2) right brachiocephalic vein (3) left brachiocephalic vein (4) confluence of inferior thyroid veins (5) inferior thyroid vein (6) middle thyroid vein (7) internal jugular vein (8) superior thyroid vein

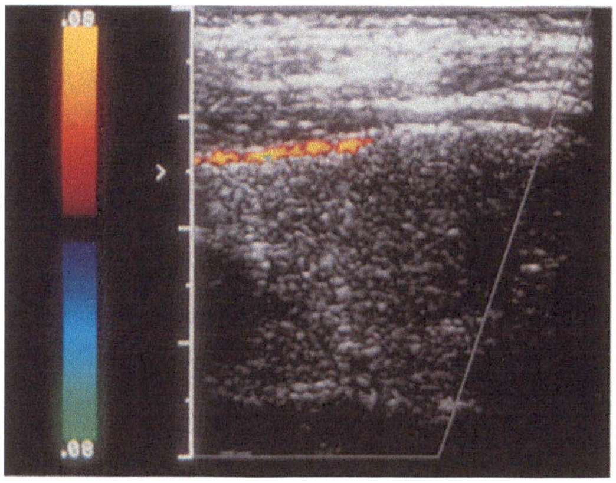

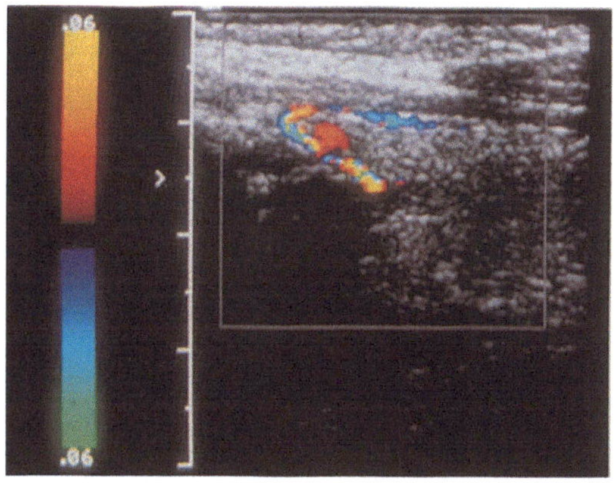

Fig. 2. (left) Normal thyroid lobe in longitudinal section: CCDS readily demonstrates the vascular plexus at the surface of the gland (red)

Fig. 3. (right) The feeding arteries and draining veins normally accumulate at the poles of the thyroid lobes (this example shows the vessels at the upper pole in longitudinal section); this normal aggregate of vessels must not be confused with a hypervascular pathologic mass (see text)

technique only rarely demonstrates normal vessels within the glandular tissue; when a segment of a vessel is noted it usually represents one of the largest supplying branches. When CCDS technique is employed many more intraglandular vessels can be identified (Fig. 4). Even with CCDS the degree of vascularization is normally not very impressive as compared to other organs such as the kidney. Relatively few vascular structures are normally shown centrally in the thyroid lobes, with a few larger vessels shown longitudinally in the periphery. Most of the vessels normally shown within the thyroid gland are veins, as can be confirmed by pulsed Doppler evaluation with spectrum analysis (Fig. 5). Spectral analysis of the major thyroid arterial channels reveals a relatively high diastolic blood flow velocity (Fig. 6).

Neither conventional gray scale ultrasound nor CCDS will give satisfactory visualization of the normal parathyroid glands; later in the chapter the role of CCDS and duplex Doppler sonography in the identification of parathyroid adenomas will be considered.

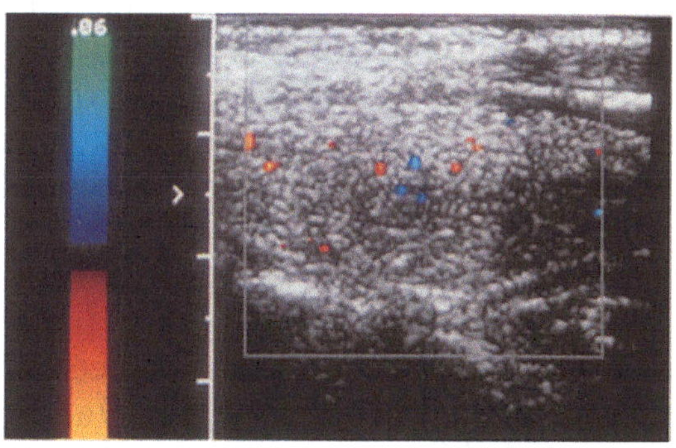

Fig. 4. Longitudinal section of normal thyroid lobe. Small intraglandular vessels are depicted by color. They are not visible in the B-mode gray scale image

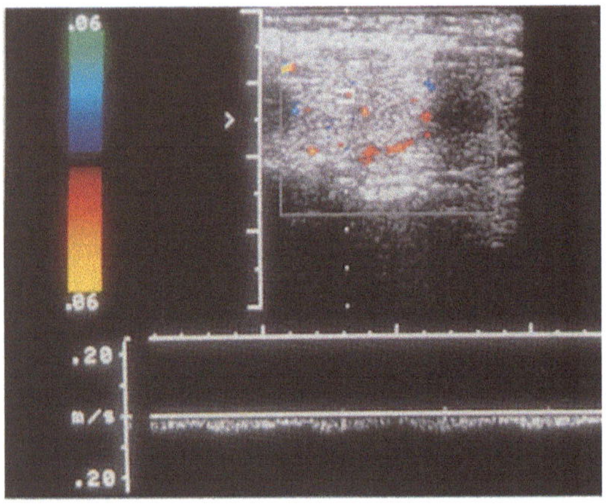

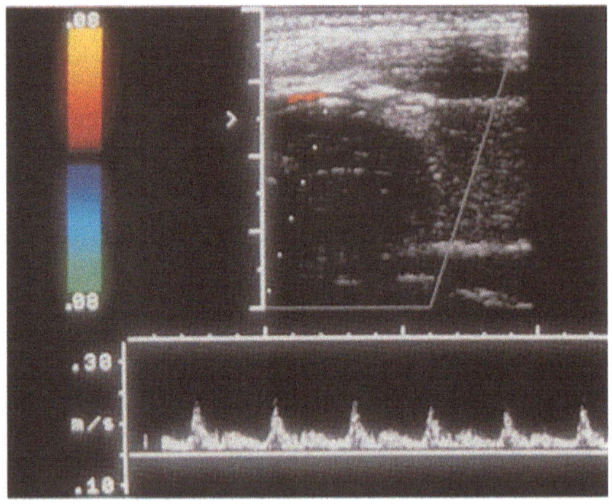

Fig. 5. (left) Most of the vessels normally shown within the thyroid gland are veins, as indicated here by pulsed Doppler evaluation with spectral waveform display

Fig. 6. (right) Examination of the superior thyroid artery: note the (normal) relatively high diastolic blood flow

Pathologic findings

1. Thyroid adenoma

An adenoma is a benign neoplastic thyroid lesion which has the potential for both increase in size and possible malignant transformation. Adenomas present as solitary or multiple nodules which can have high, low, or intermediate echogenicity and which are surrounded in most cases by some normal thyroid parenchyma. As a rule they are well demarcated from adjacent glandular tissue and may show what has been referred to as the "halo sign": a thin hypoechogenic margin completely encircling the nodule (Fig. 7a). CCDS often demonstrates hypervascularity within this hypoechogenic region (Fig. 7b).

As a rule, simple thyroid adenomas show no evidence of central hypervascularization. *Autonomous* adenomas, on the other hand, are well documented in the literature to have both central and peripheral hypervascularization (Fig. 8a, b). When this type of pattern is shown by CCDS, radionuclide imaging (eventually to include a suppression test) should be carried out to help establish the diagnosis. According to the literature, differential diagnosis of a hypervascular thyroid nodule includes thyroid carcinoma (see below). Simple, non-autonomous thyroid adenomas can also show evidence of central vascularization in some cases; it is therefore necessary to carry out radionuclide imaging and follow up low-uptake lesions with needle puncture or biopsy. And, as will be emphasized below, *absent* central hypervascularity does not necessarily rule out malignancy.

Since the gray scale ultrasound findings are also inadequate for reliable determination of whether a nodule is benign or malignant, those having low tracer uptake by nuclear medicine imaging (which are at risk for malignancy, especially when they are solitary) should undergo needle biopsy or surgery (Fig. 9a, b). Lesions with cystic components (Fig. 10) are regarded by some authors as having a low risk for malignancy, but it must be noted that almost one third of papillary

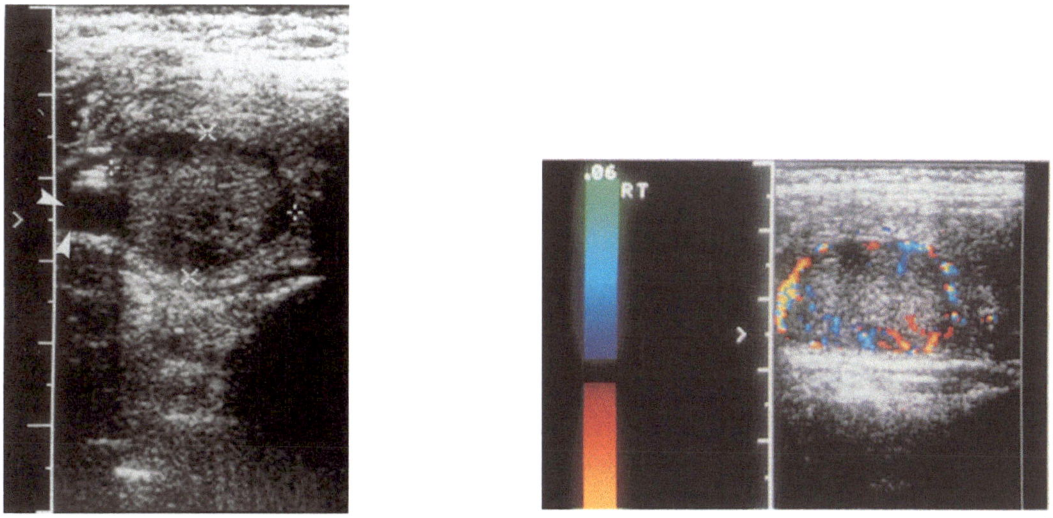

a *b*

Fig. 7a. Gray scale ultrasound image of a follicular adenoma within the right lobe of the thyroid gland (arrowheads = common carotid artery). The nodule is encircled by a thin hypoechogenic margin, the so-called "halo"

Fig. 7b. CCDS of the same lesion as in Fig. 7a, but in longitudinal section: the halo proves to be hypervascular. The vessels surround the nodule completely. Within the nodule no hypervascularity is demonstrated

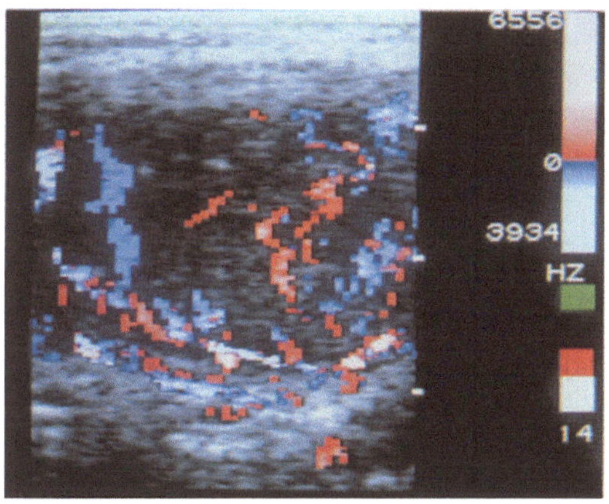

Fig. 8. CCDS of an autonomous adenoma: there is marked increase in vascularity in the center of the lesion as well as at the periphery

carcinomas will have associated cystic changes. Hyperechogenic nodules without evidence of local invasion or adjacent lymphadenopathy are usually low-risk lesions.

2. Thyroid carcinoma

Carcinomas are, by definition, malignant tumors of epithelial cell origin. Histologically the thyroid carcinomas can be divided into four types: follicular, papillary,

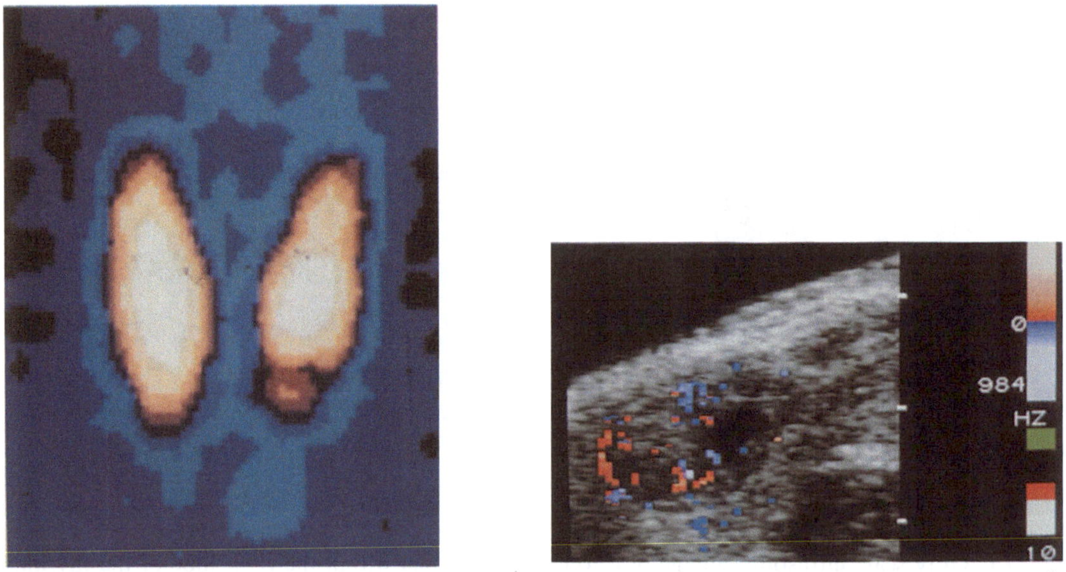

a *b*

Fig. 9a. Radionuclide imaging shows a low-uptake lesion at the lower pole of the left thyroid lobe. The rest of the gland is normal

Fig. 9b. CCDS of the low uptake lesion shown in Fig. 9a: there is an inhomogeneous nodule with a hypervascular CCDS pattern. Histology of the operative specimen showed nests of papillary carcinoma within the nodule

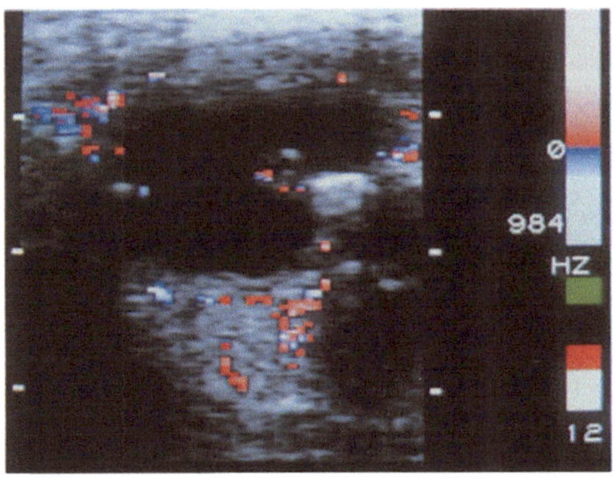

Fig. 10. CCDS of an adenoma with degenerative changes including a cystic component. Histology showed no signs of malignancy in this lesion

Table 1. CCDS features of thyroid carcinoma (from the authors' own investigations)

Type	N	Central hypervasc.	Peripheral hypervasc.	Central and peripheral hypervasc.
Papillary carcinoma	13	5 (38%)	3 (23%)	4 (31%)
Follicular carcinoma	5	–	3 (60%)	–
Anaplastic carcinoma	3	1 (33%)	–	–

anaplastic and medullary. Anaplastic carcinoma has a tendency to early invasion of surrounding structures, a feature which may be evident sonographically and is one of the few reliable signs of malignancy. The presence of cervical lymphadenopathy should also lead to the consideration of malignancy in the thyroid gland. Unfortunately, there are no other sonomorphological signs of malignancy which do not have significant overlap with findings in benign lesions. It had been hoped that CCDS might help to overcome this limitation by providing additional information which could better differentiate malignant from benign masses. An early hypothesis that thyroid carcinomas should be hypervascular seemed to have some support in initial reports in the literature, but in our experience a high number of proven carcinomas showed no evidence of increased vascularity centrally. Some of these even resembled adenomas, having a ring of vessels at the periphery of the lesion (Table 1). We have found that thyroid carcinomas can present with a rather wide variety of sonomorphological and vascular patterns (Figs. 11–15).

3. Other malignant lesions

Non-epithelial malignant tumors are of secondary importance in the thyroid gland but do deserve mention. Malignant hemangioendothelioma is a sarcoma of the thyroid gland which has been well described pathologically but has not yet been characterized by CCDS; this is also true for fibrosarcoma of the thyroid gland.

We have examined several malignant lymphomas of the non-Hodgkin type using CCDS. All of these were hypoechogenic relative to normal thyroid tissue and showed no "halo". The degree of vascularization visible using CCDS was generally low, with even fewer vessels shown within the lesion than in the normal portions of the gland. In some cases the margins of the lesion were well defined (Fig. 16) while in other cases there was infiltration of almost the entire lobe of the thyroid gland and ill-defined lesion borders (Fig. 17). These results must be considered only preliminary until a larger series of cases can be evaluated.

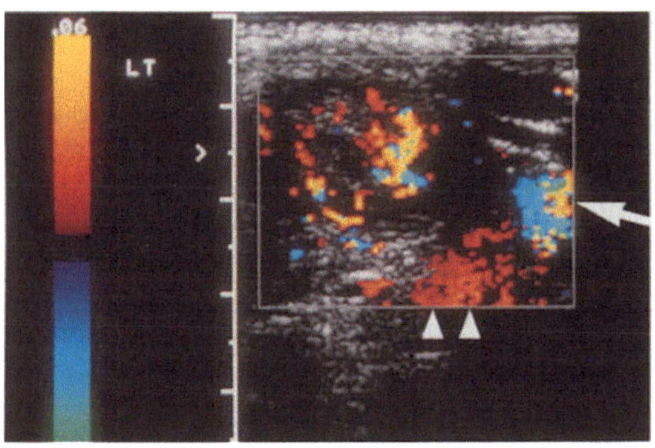

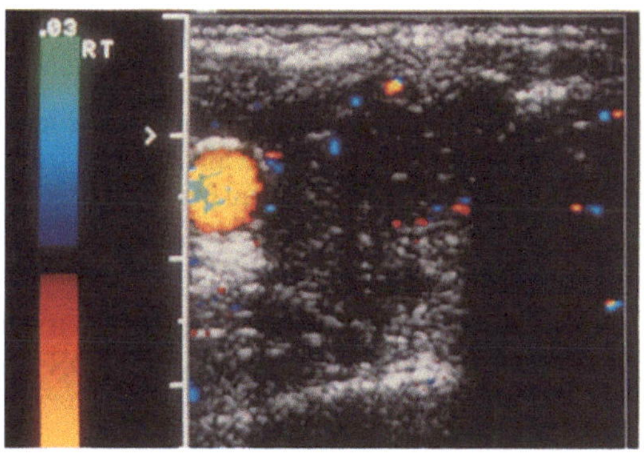

Fig. 11. (left) Papillary carcinoma in the left thyroid lobe (arrow = carotid artery, arrowheads = motion artifacts). The lesion is clearly hypervascular. This pattern can be observed in many carcinomas, as well as in autonomous adenomas

Fig. 12. (right) Papillary carcinoma with invasion of lymph vessels (right thyroid lobe, transverse section): in contrast to the lesion shown in Fig. 11, no increased vascularity is demonstrated (carotid artery shown in red)

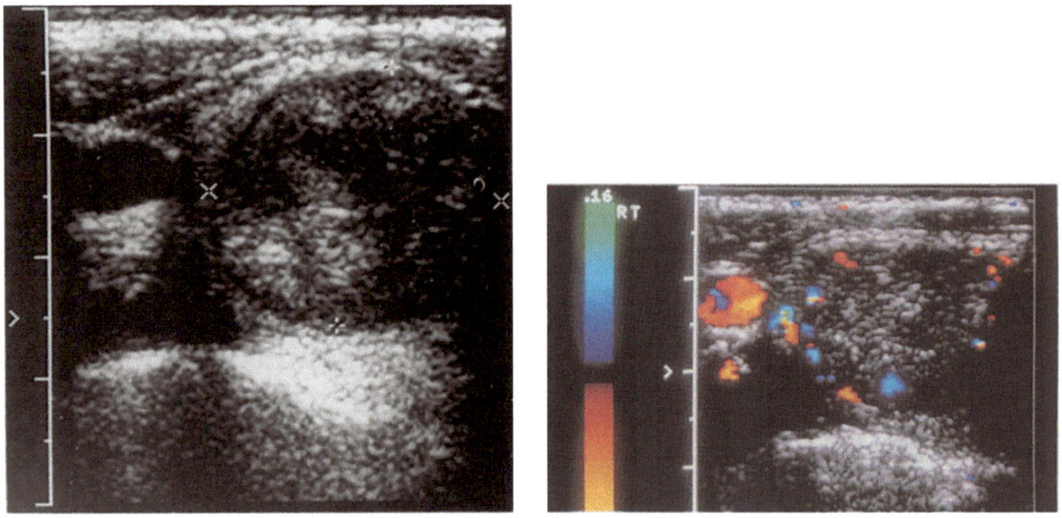

a *b*

Fig. 13. Gray scale ultrasound scan ***a*** and corresponding CCDS image ***b*** of a papillary carcinoma in the right thyroid lobe (transverse section, carotid artery shown in red on CCDS image). Note the similarity of the findings to those shown for the adenoma in Fig. 7a, b including a "halo" on the gray scale scan

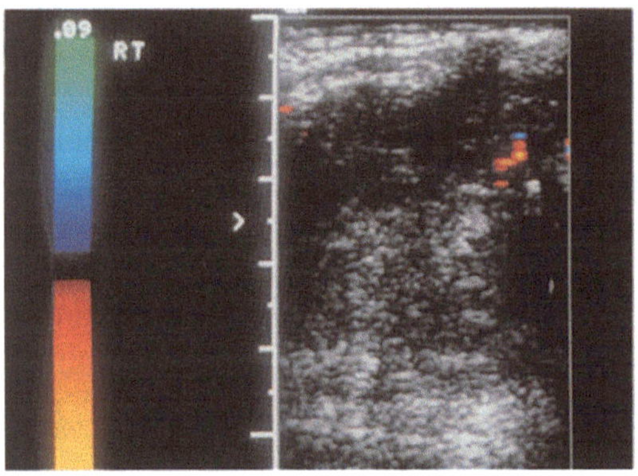

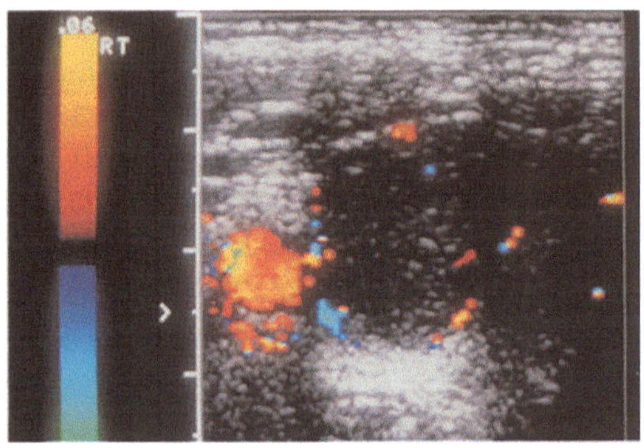

Fig. 14. (left) This anaplastic carcinoma shows nearly no internal vascularization on the CCDS image, but the gray scale characteristics of inhomogeneity of structure and ill-defined border segments suggest a malignant lesion

Fig. 15. (right) Follicular carcinoma shown in a transverse section through the right thyroid lobe (CCA shown in red). In our small series of five cases (see Table 1) none had evidence of increased central vascularity; 3 of the 5 had evidence of some vessels at the periphery as illustrated in this figure

Metastatic malignant lesions in the thyroid gland are rare, so it is not surprising that as yet no reports of their CCDS characteristics have been published.

4. Goiter

The diagnostic value of CCDS in goiter has not yet been determined. Our initial experience has been that CCDS does not add any diagnostic information except in cases where there is evidence of a hypervascular nodule (which should then be

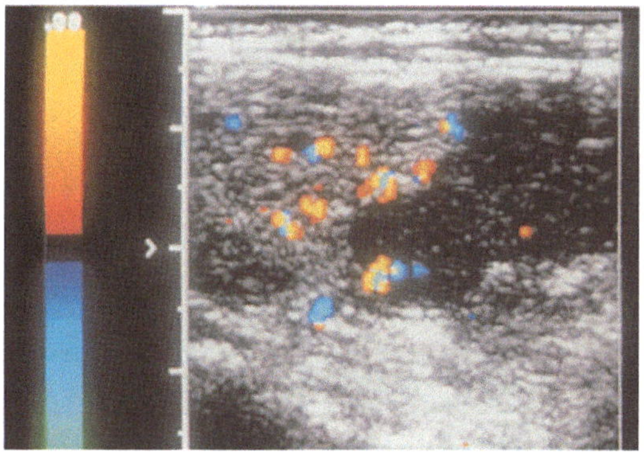

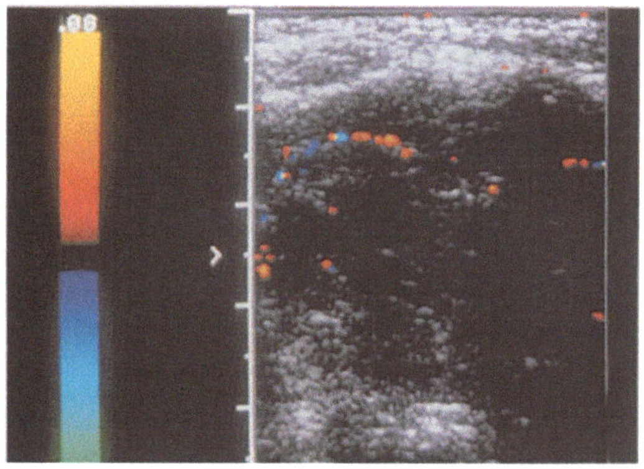

Fig. 16. (left) Malignant non-Hodgkin lymphoma of the thyroid gland. There is a hypoechogenic, well defined lesion at the lower pole of the left lobe. Within the lesion, there are even fewer vessels seen than in the normal parts of the gland

Fig. 17. (right) Maligant non-Hodgkin lymphoma of the thyroid gland. The lesion somewhat resembles the anaplastic carcinoma shown in Fig. 14. It shows only minimal central vascularization

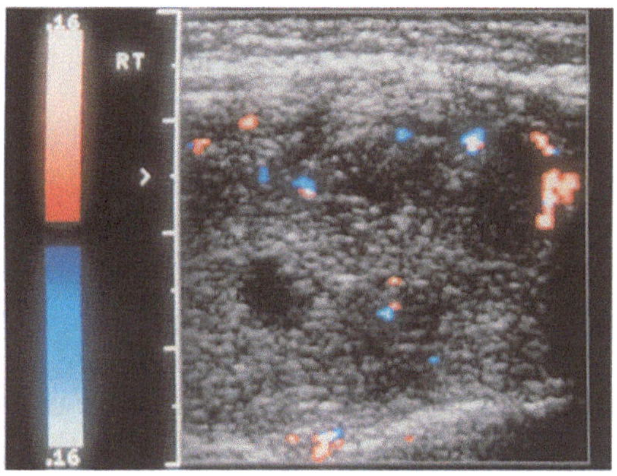

Fig. 18. In this goiter several nodules are visible. The pattern of vascularization is nonspecific

further evaluated by radionuclide imaging). Often there is minimal vascularization noted in the central portion of nodular parenchymal areas; marked hypervascularization is usually not encountered (Fig. 18).

5. Thyroiditis

Thyroiditis can be subdivided into acute, subacute and chronic forms. Histological findings can include inflammatory granulomas (subacute thyroiditis of de Quervain), infiltration by lymphocytes and plasma cells (thyroiditis lymphomatosa of Hashimoto) or extensive fibrosis (ligneous goiter of Riedel). These aseptic subacute or chronic inflammatory processes must be differentiated from acute purulent thyroiditis secondary to septicemia, which is less common.

From a sonographic standpoint, thyroiditis is most commonly associated with gland enlargement and hypoechogenic areas. These sonomorphological changes may affect the entire gland or just portions of it. CCDS may show marked hyper-

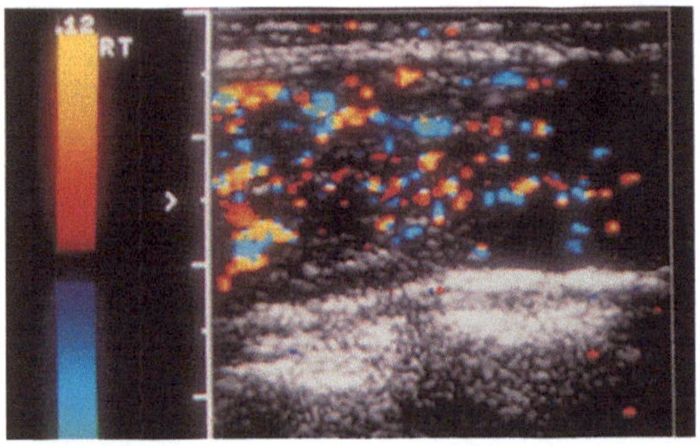

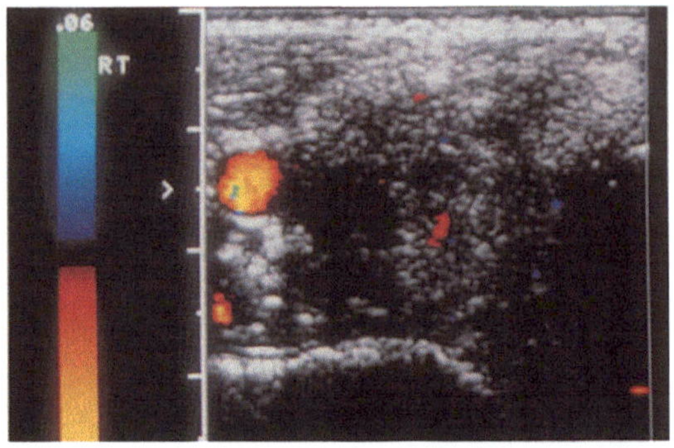

Fig. 19. (left) Hashimoto's thyroiditis with a striking degree of increased vascularity; the same pattern was shown in the other thyroid lobe and is suggestive of inflammatory changes in the gland. Gray scale imaging showed generalized hypoechogenicity

Fig. 20. (right) Granulomatous thyroiditis: comparison with Figs. 14 and 17 will illustrate how difficult it would be to differentiate this lesion from malignant masses

vascularization in the diffusely affected areas (Fig. 19). Nodular structures may be present within the thyroid tissue, in which case differentiation from carcinoma is difficult (Fig. 20).

6. Basedow's or Graves' Disease

Exophthalmic goiter, referred to as Basedow's Disease or Graves' Disease (after the German and Irish physicians Carl A. von Basedow and Robert James Graves, respectively, who described the disorder in the mid-1800's), is characterized by clinical symptoms related to thyrotoxicosis (hyperthyroidism). The diagnosis usually is confirmed by laboratory tests and radionuclide imaging. In recent years there have been reports of a typical vascularization pattern within the thyroid gland in Graves disease. Referred to as "thyroid inferno", it is characterized by pulsatile hypervascularization (Fig. 21). High flow velocities are present in systole, with much lower or even absent flow during diastole. It is this pulsatile or "high-resis-

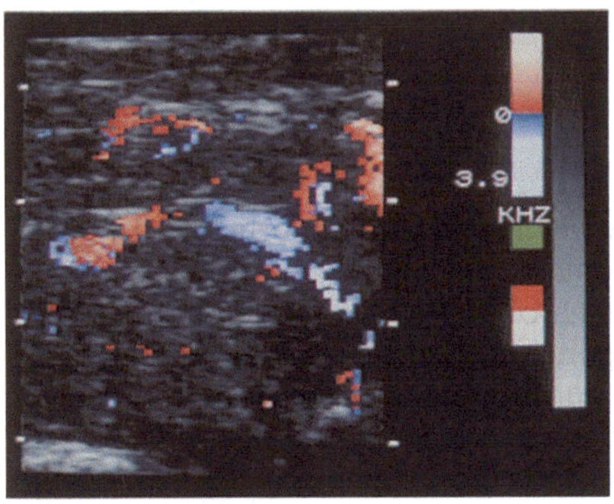

Fig. 21. Appearance of thyroid gland in Graves' disease: typical pattern of "thyroid inferno" with hypervascularization (and marked pulsatility noted when viewed in real time)

tance" pattern which differentiates Graves disease from the more continuous flow pattern throughout the cardiac cycle seen in other conditions such as thyroiditis. With treatment the vascularization pattern returns to normal.

7. Iodine-induced changes of blood flow

The fact that thyroid blood supply can be decreased by iodine administration has been known since the initial descriptive work by the American physician Henry S. Plummer early in this century. Many surgeons still insist on preoperative administration of iodine because of this effect. The role of prophylactic intake of iodine in the prevention of accumulation of radioactive iodine isotopes in the thyroid gland following nuclear accidents may also be based in part on the Wolff-Chaikoff effect which involves some sort of iodine-induced autoregulation of blood supply.

We have been able to demonstrate a marked decrease of CCDS-detected blood flow in the thyroid gland in patients undergoing angiography (Fig. 22a, b). In this study the administration of non-ionic contrast material resulted in extremely high serum concentrations of iodine (protein-bound iodine and total iodine serum concentration) after the angiographic procedure; iodine levels returned to normal about a week later. CCDS evidence of vascularization of the thyroid gland correlated well with iodine levels, showing diminished flow within one day after angiography and a return to pre-angiographic levels one week later.

8. Parathyroid adenoma

The parathyroid glands are most commonly located along the dorsal surface of the thyroid gland, although some patients may have atypically positioned parathyroid

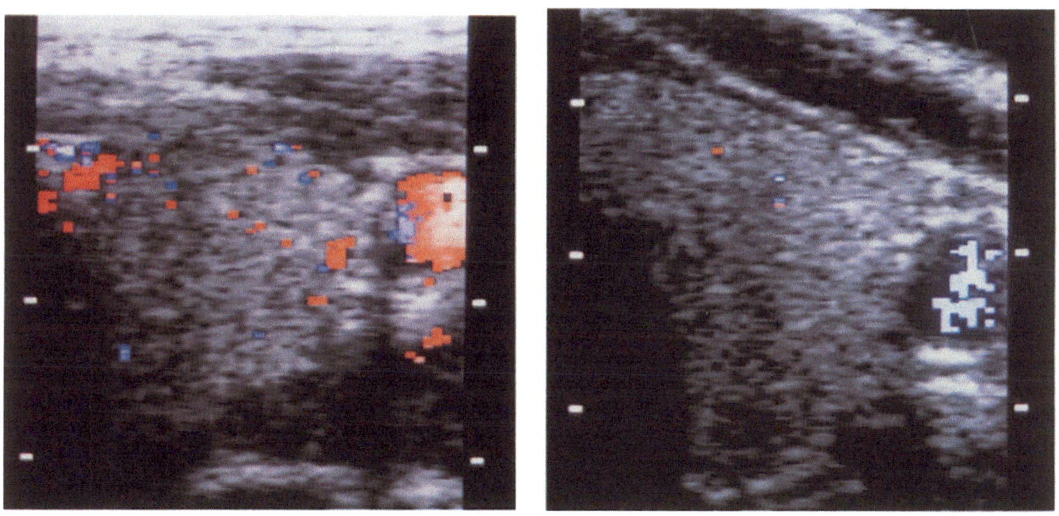

a *b*

Fig. 22a. CCDS image of normal vascular pattern of the thyroid gland before iodine loaded

Fig. 22b. Reduced vascularity of the thyroid gland one day after iodine load (angiography with 130 ml of contrast medium containing 300 mg iodine per ml)

tissue in locations such as the mediastinum. In 90% of cadavars there are four parathyroid glands. About 80% of patients with primary hyperparathyroidism will have evidence of a parathyroid adenoma, 13% will have hyperplasia of all the parathyroid glands, and a small percentage will have underlying parathyroid carcinoma. In addition to the typical laboratory findings of hypercalcemia, hypophosphatemia, and elevated plasma levels of PTH, there are also typical radiographic skeletal changes such as subperiosteal and endosteal bone resorption in the phalanges of the hand (Fig. 23).

When an adenoma of a parathyroid gland is suspected, sonography is indicated for preoperative identification of the enlarged gland. While normal parathyroid glands are not generally identified by sonography, a sensitivity of up to 85% is reported for identification of adenomas. They usually present as homogeneous, hypoechoic oval-shaped nodules, often along the medial border of the mid-to-lower portion of a thyroid lobe. Parathyroid adenomas arising in atypical locations are, in contrast, difficult or impossible to detect by sonography.

Within parathyroid adenomas duplex Doppler sonography will show characteristic flow patterns (Fig. 24a, b). CCDS readily demonstrates a hypervascular pattern (Fig. 25). The identification of a hypervascular nodule in the expected location of one of the parathyroid glands, in conjunction with clinical and radiological signs of hyperparathyroidism, suggests a high likelihood of parathyroid adenoma. If typical laboratory and bone-related changes are absent, however, the differential diagnosis must include *thyroid* adenoma or carcinoma (see above).

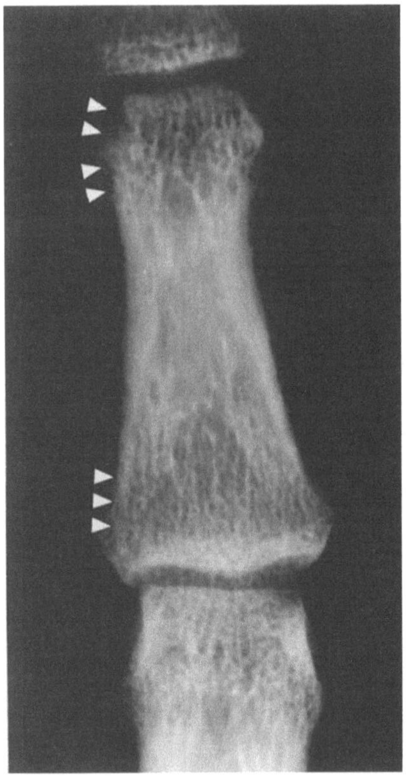

Fig. 23. Magnification radiograph of the phalanges of the hand: subperiosteal bone resorption is noted (arrowheads) consistent with abnormal bone loss in this patient with primary hyperparathyroidism

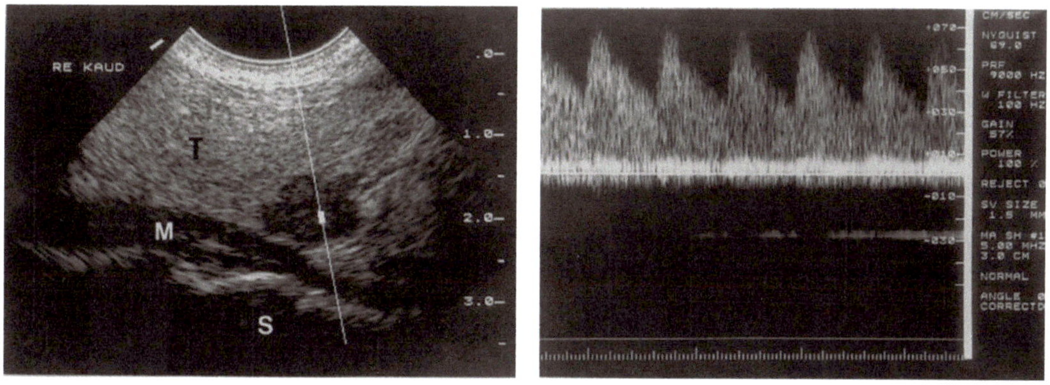

a *b*

Fig. 24 ***a***, ***b***. Typical appearance of parathyroid adenoma in a patient with primary hyperparathyroidism. There is a hypoechogenic nodule in the parathyroid region, in which arterial Doppler signals with high diastolic flow velocity can be recorded. (T = thyroid gland, M = longus colli muscle, S = cervical spine)

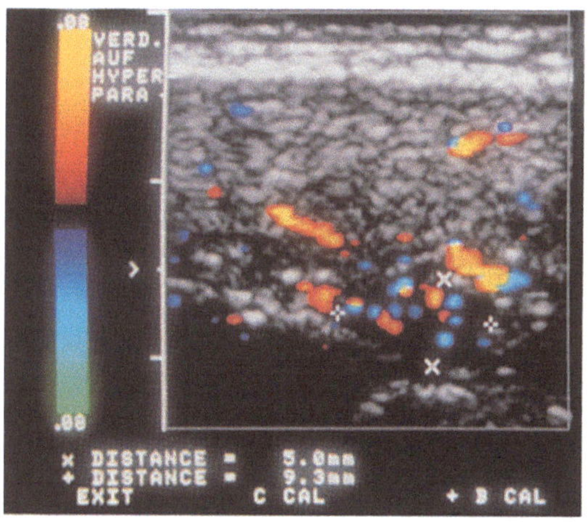

Fig. 25. CCDS can readily demonstrate the hypervascular pattern in parathyroid adenomas (the lesion is demarcated by the measurement caliper marks)

Conclusion

CCDS adds significantly to the ultrasound evaluation of thyroid pathology by demonstration of thyroid arteries and veins and visualization of small vessels within normal or abnormal glandular structures. The increased vascularity typically associated with parathyroid adenomas can also be documented by CCDS. However, the exact role of CCDS techniques in thyroid and parathyroid pathology will only become fully understood as more extensive experience is gained in correlating CCDS patterns with histologic findings, especially in the case of the less commonly encountered types of malignancy.

References

Cole-Beuglet C, Goldberg BB (1983) New high-resolution ultrasound evaluation of diseases of the thyroid gland. A review article. JAMA 149:2941–2944

Czembirek H, Tscholakoff D, Gritzmann N (1988) Sonographie der Schilddrüse. In: Czembirek H, Frühwald F, Gritzmann N (Hrsg) Kopf-Hals-Sonographie. Springer, Wien New York, S 189–201

Dwarakanathan AA, Saclarides TJ, Witt TR, Ryan WG, Kath JM, Mesleh GF, Economu SG (1986) The role of ultrasonography in the evaluation of primary hyperparathyroidism. J Surg Gyn Obstet 163:504–508

Fobbe F, Wolf KJ (1988) Erste klinische Erfahrungen mit der Angiodynographie. Fortschr Röntgenstr 148:259–264

Fobbe F, Finke R, Reichenstein E, Schleusener H, Wolf KJ (1989) Appearance of thyroid diseases using colour-coded duplex sonography. Eur J Radiol 9:29–31

Gorman B, Charboneau JW, James EM, Reading CC, World LE, Graut CS, Gharib H, Hay ID (1987) Medullary thyroid carcinoma: Role of high-resolution ultrasound. Radiology 147–150

Gritzmann N (1988) Nebenschilddrüsen. In: Czembirek H, Frühwald F, Gritzmann N (Hrsg) Kopf-Hals-Sonographie. Springer, Wien New York, S 202–210

Hayashi Y, Misaki T, Iida Y, Kasagi K, Endo K, Konishi J, Torizuka K, Mori T, Makimoto K (1986) Real-time ultrasonography of thyroid nodules. Acta Radiol Diagn 27:403–408

Hübsch P, Niederle B, Barton P, Pesau B, Knittel M, Schratter M, Hermann M, Längle F (1992) Farbkodierte Dopplersonographie der Schilddrüse: Ein Fortschritt in der Karzinomdiagnostik? Fortschr Röntgenstr (im Druck)

Katz JF, Kane RA, Reyes J, Clarke MP, Hill TC (1984) Thyroid nodules: sonographic-pathologic correlation. Radiology 151:741–745

Moreau JF (1983) Parathyroid glands. In: Bruneton IN (ed) Ultrasonography of the neck. Springer, Berlin Heidelberg New York Tokyo

Pfannenstiel P, Baew-Christow Th (1985) Röntgen-Computertomographie und Sonographie in der Schilddrüsendiagnostik. Zentralblatt für Chirurgie 110:1105–1114

Pristautz H, Petritsch W, Schreiber F, Warnkross H, Pietsch B, Passath A, Leb G, Tilz P, Kellner A (1989) Sonographie und Zytologie bei kalten Schilddrüsenknoten. Fortschr Röntgenstr 150:250–254

Ralls PW, Mayekawa DS, Lee KP, Colletti PM, Radin DR, Boswell WD, Halls JM (1988) Color-flow Doppler sonography in Graves disease: "Thyroid inferno". AJR 150:781–784

Sample WF, Mitchel SP, Bledsoe RC (1978) Parathyroid ultrasonography. Radiology 127:485

Scheible W, Leopold GR, Woo VL, Gosink BB (1979) High resolution real-time ultrasonography of thyroid nodules. Radiology 133:413–417

Schneider K (1991) Sonographic imaging of the thyroid in children. Prog Pediatr Surg 26:1–14

Schwaighofer B, Kurtaran A, Hübsch P, Frühwald F, Barton P, Trattnig S (1988) Farbkodierte Dopplersonographie bei Schilddrüsenerkrankungen: erste Erfahrungen. Fortschr Röntgenstr 149:310–313

Scink J, Schober O (1989) Die Sonographie der Schilddrüse. Radiologe 29:95–102

Simeone JF, Daniels GH, Mueller PR, Maloof F, van Sonnenberg E, Hall DA, O'Connel RS, Ferucci JT Jr, Wittenberg J (1982) High resolution real time sonography of the thyroid. Radiology 145:431–435

Solbiati L, Volterrani L, Rizzatto G, Bazzocchi M, Busilacchi P, Candiani F, Ferrari F, Giuseppetti G, Maresca G, Mirk P, Rubaltelli L, Zappasodi F (1985) The thyroid gland with low uptake lesions: evaluation by ultrasound. Radiology 155:187–191

Thomas Chr, Bautz W, Müller-Schauenburg W, Feine U (1989) Angiodynographie bei umschriebenen Schilddrüsenveränderungen. Fortschr Röntgenstr 150:72–75

Tscholakoff D, Grubeck-Leobenstein B, Czembirek H, Haller J, Leitner H (1985) Sonographie der Schilddrüse mit hochauflösenden real-time Geräten. Fortschr Röntgenstr 142:309–313

Weissel M, Hübsch P, Kurtaran A, Kainz H, Frühwald F (1990) In-vivo evidence for iodine-induced decrease of thyroid blood flow by color coded Doppler sonography in normal human thyroid glands. Acta Medica Austriaca Sonderheft 17:64–65

7
Color-coded Doppler sonography of the veins of the neck and upper extremities

P. Hübsch and S. Trattnig

Introduction

The cervical veins can be divided into superficial and deep veins with respect to their position relative to the deep cervical fascia. The superficial veins drain the blood mostly to the external jugular vein. The internal jugular vein (IJV), which is the largest vein in the neck, receives blood from the sigmoid sinus, skull, face and a large portion of the neck (Fig. 1). The IJV is easily assessed sonographically, descending lateral to the internal and common carotid arteries to its junction with the brachiocephalic vein. Only the most cranial portion of the vein, including the superior bulb, cannot be sonographically visualized; the inferior bulb is readily demonstrated in most cases. Because of the clinical importance of the IJV, this vessel deserves special attention during sonographic evaluation of the neck.

The subclavian veins can also be examined sonographically, but complete visualization of the brachiocephalic veins is limited due to partial superposition of bony structures (clavicle and sternum) (Fig. 2). This is more of a problem for the left brachiocephalic vein due to its length (more than twice as long as the right brachiocephalic vein) as it courses from left to right deep to the manubrium of the sternum. Even with these limitations, sonography (and especially CCDS) has proven to be useful for the examination of the subclavian and upper limb veins. This chapter focuses on the normal appearance of the veins of the neck and upper extremities, and on the most common pathologic findings, thrombosis and involvement with metastatic tumor.

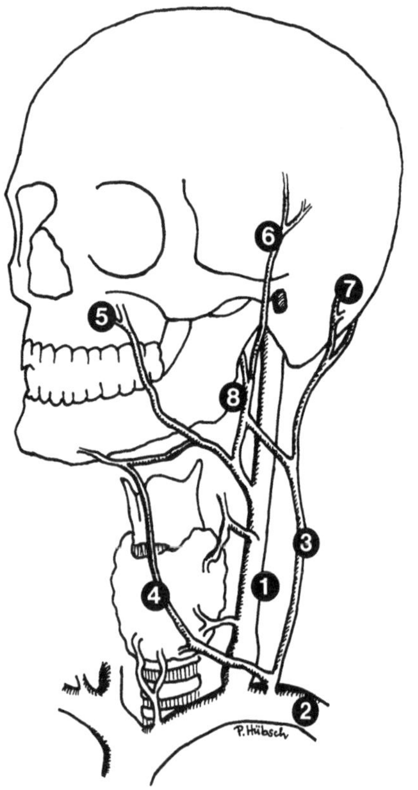

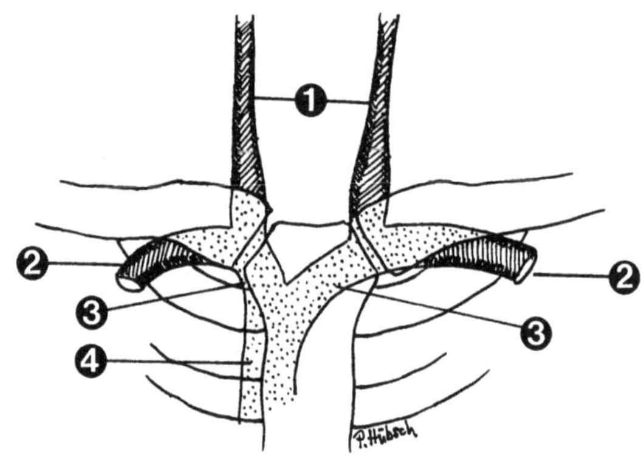

Fig. 1. (left) Synopsis of major cervical veins: (1) internal jugular vein (2) subclavian vein, (3) external jugular vein, (4) anterior jugular vein, (5) facial vein, (6) superficial temporal vein, (7) occipital vein, (8) retromandibular vein. The vertebral venous plexus is not shown in this illustration

Fig. 2. (right) Major veins of the thoracic inlet: (1) internal jugular veins, (2) subclavian veins, (3) brachiocephalic veins, (4) superior vena cava. The dotted parts of the veins are not visible directly by using ultrasound because of overlying bony structures and/or lung

Examination technique

Generally the patient is examined in the supine position; for the examination of the IJV the head is rotated slightly back and to the opposite side. The IJV is easily found lateral to the carotid arteries. On the left side, the caudal part of the vein often overlaps the common carotid artery. All parts of the vein must be examined in longitudinal and transverse planes. In many patients when a linear scanhead is used, the inferior bulb of the vessel can only be seen in an angled transverse section because of acoustic shadowing caused by the clavicle. This angled transverse approach also allows visualization of the proximal portion of both brachiocephalic veins in most patients. The subclavian vein can be evaluated by using an infraclavicular approach and identifying the vein as it runs parallel to the subclavian artery.

Examination of the veins of the upper limb is facilitated by using related anatomic landmarks such as the clavicle, muscles, and arteries to help in the identification of the course of the major veins (cephalic, basilic, brachial, axillary, and subclavian). Scan technique is important, especially with regard to the amount of pressure exerted. The internal jugular vein and many veins of the upper extremity are superficially positioned and can be compressed if excessive transducer pressure is used; this can lead to incorrect interpretation of the study. However, if pressure is deliberately applied as a form of "sonopalpation" this can actually help to differentiate veins with normal lumens from those containing thrombus (see section 1 under "Pathologic findings" below). The examination should not be limited to a single vein but should include all major tributaries as well as the contralateral veins for comparison. Pulsed Doppler waveform tracings for velocity measurement should be obtained routinely in addition to the color-coded Doppler findings. Color sensitivity settings may have to be individually optimized for the particular vein being evaluated (for example, rather high flow velocities may be encountered in the internal jugular vein).

Normal findings

In contrast to the arteries, veins have a thin, highly echogenic wall without layers. The lumen of the vein is usually anechoic in the gray-scale image; occasionally moving echoes can be shown within the lumen, especially in areas of turbulence. Distension during the Valsalva maneuver can be seen in the normal IJV and, to a lesser degree, in the subclavian vein. The IJV is normally wider in the lower one-third of the neck than in its more cranial portion. Slight turbulence, seen as a mixture of colors near the inferior bulb, is a common finding in normal cases (Fig. 3); the more cranial portion of the IJV shows mostly a laminar flow pattern (Fig. 4). A valve can be seen in the inferior bulb area in most patients; it is usually best visualized on the B-mode portion of the examination since it is often obscured by superimposed color on CCDS. Brownlow, Dresser and McKinney suggest that the importance of this jugular valve has been underestimated. They note that the valve can be rendered incompetent by damage from catheterization, chronic tricuspid valve regurgitation, or sustained periods of increased central venous pressure

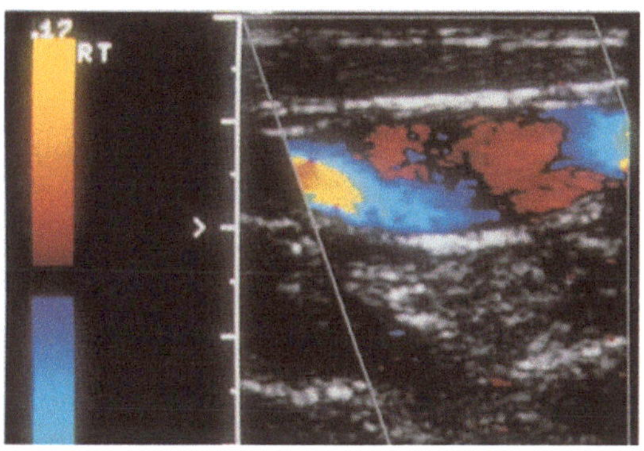

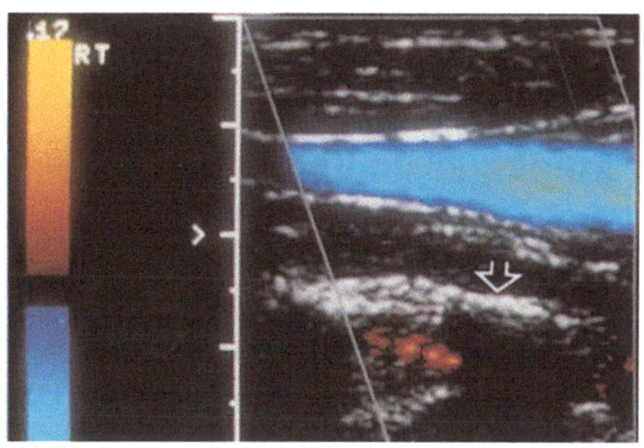

Fig. 3. (left) CCDS of inferior bulb of a normal internal jugular vein (longitudinal section): Turbulence related to flow deceleration in the widened lumen is common in this part of the vessel and is indicated by a variety of colors

Fig. 4. (right) Superior part of a normal IJV (longitudinal section): In this region the blood flow usually is laminar, which is indicated by higher blood flow velocities in the center of the vessel (light blue) and relatively low blood flow velocity near the vessel wall (dark blue). Deep to the vein, the vertebral artery is visible (red). The echogenic line (arrow) with dorsal shadowing represents the surface of a transverse process of a cervical vertebra

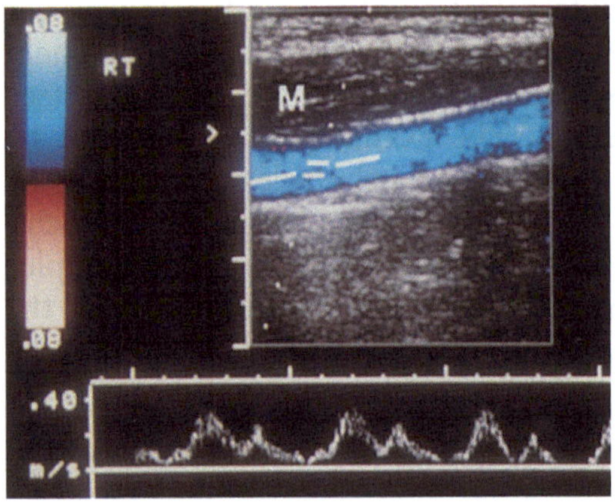

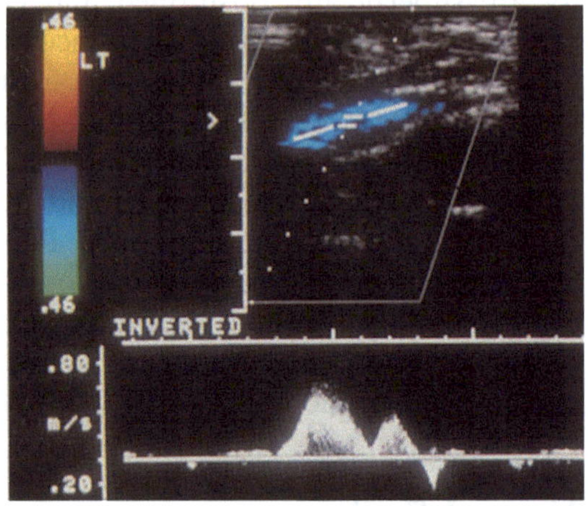

a *b*

Fig. 5a. Normal IJV with Doppler spectrum (M = sternocleidomastoid muscle): alternating accelerations and decelerations of blood flow velocity are related to cardiac dynamics (see text for details)

Fig. 5b. The same blood flow velocity pattern as in the IJV can be observed in the subclavian vein

due to positive end-expiratory pressure (PEEP) respirator settings. The increased back-pressure in the IJV may lead to cerebral venous congestion and the so-called "brain-respirator syndrome" with confusion and other symptoms of cerebral dysfunction. The authors suggest a possible role for Doppler ultrasound in the screening of patients for incompetence of the internal jugular vein valve prior to extended use of respirator support.

Veins of the thoracic outlet and their direct tributaries have characteristic Doppler waveform patterns related to the close relationship of these veins to the heart. Alternating accelerations and decelerations of blood flow velocity (Fig. 5a, b) are seen; the first of the two adjacent velocity peaks is related to atrial pressure changes during ventricular systole while the second peak is caused by opening of the tricuspid valve. These cyclic flow velocity changes are easily observed in real time with CCDS and have a role to play in the indirect diagnosis of thrombosis, as will be further discussed in the next section.

Pathologic findings

1. Thrombosis

Thrombosis of the IJV and subclavian vein can occur in association with prolonged venous compression, inflammatory conditions, neoplastic disease, surgery, heart disease, and intravenous drug abuse. Another common cause of thrombosis in these veins is the placement of catheters and pacemaker leads. Thrombus formation may occur as a result of damage to the vessel wall, hypotension, bacteremia, catheter coiling, or a combination of these factors. The presence of a "foreign body", namely the catheter, may also be an important factor. The risk of thrombosis generally increases directly with the length of time the catheter is in place; rarely thrombosis may occur in the vessels contralateral to the catheter site. Thrombosis of the subclavian vein can affect the internal jugular vein and vice-versa.

In most cases, thrombosis of the internal jugular vein is asymptomatic; it is, however, a potentially life-threatening condition and can in rare instances be associated with cerebral edema. The thrombosed vein may be palpable on physical examination.

Arm swelling is a consistent finding when there is thrombosis of the subclavian vein (Fig. 6); distension of the ipsilateral external jugular vein may be present as well (Fig. 7). Pulmonary embolism, which can be life-threatening, is reported to occur in up to 12% of cases of subclavian vein thrombosis.

The criteria for diagnosis of thrombosis using real-time sonography and CCDS are shown in Table 1. Old thrombus has an echogenic pattern (Fig. 8), while recent thrombus produces very few intraluminal echoes (Figs. 9, 10). When recent thrombosis is present CCDS (with maximum sensitivity settings) will show absence of color-encoding in the entire vessel or in those portions of the lumen occupied by thrombus; this technique allows identification of even small thrombi (Fig. 11 a–c).

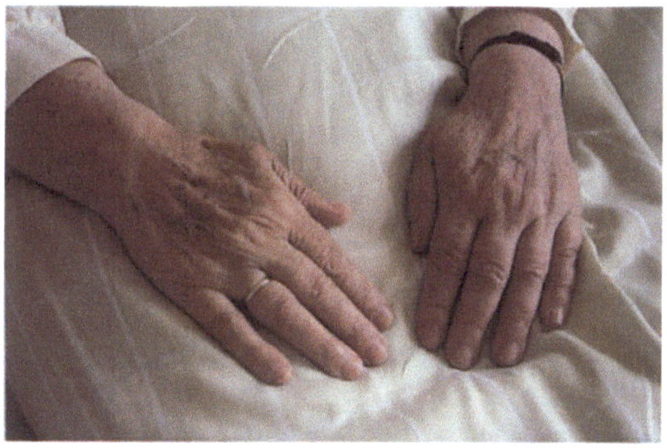

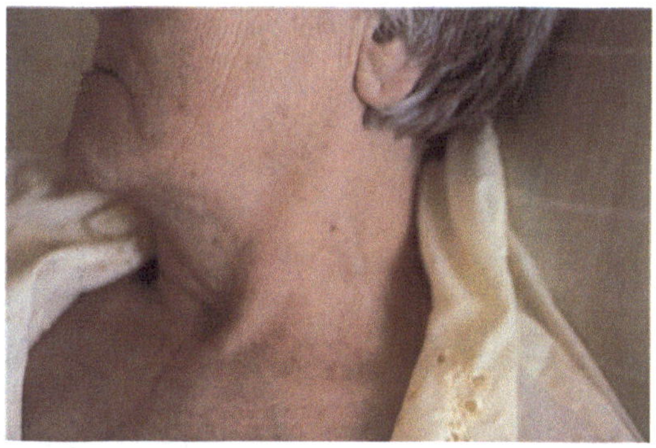

Fig. 6. (left) Swelling of the upper limb in a patient with thrombosis of the subclavian vein; note the difference between right and left side skin color

Fig. 7. (right) Distension of the external jugular vein in ipsilateral subclavian vein thrombosis (same patient as Fig. 6)

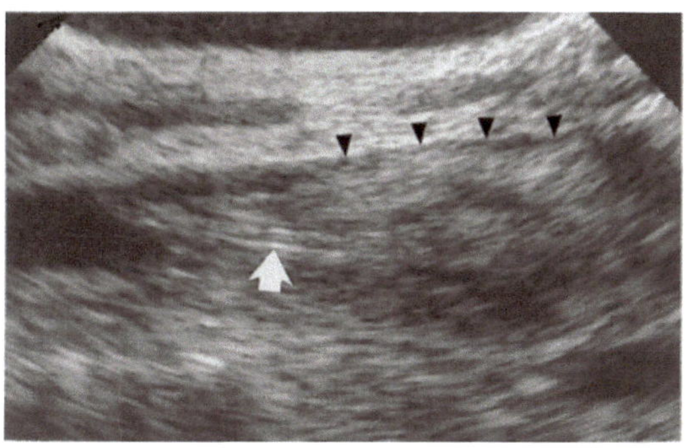

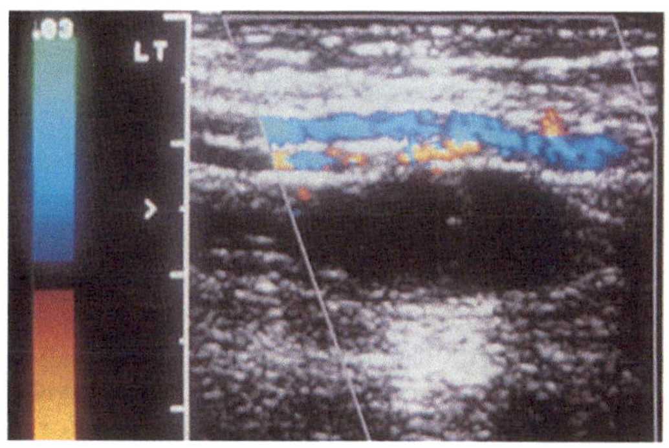

Fig. 8. (left) Longitudinal section of IJV thrombosis secondary to a central venous catheter (arrow). The echogenic thrombus (arrowheads) appears slightly inhomogeneous; the vein is distended and incompressible

Fig. 9. (right) Recent thrombosis of the IJV (longitudinal section): the lumen is nearly echo-free, but no flow signals can be recorded within the vessel; a small vein is demonstrated superficial to the IJV and may possibly represent a collateral vessel

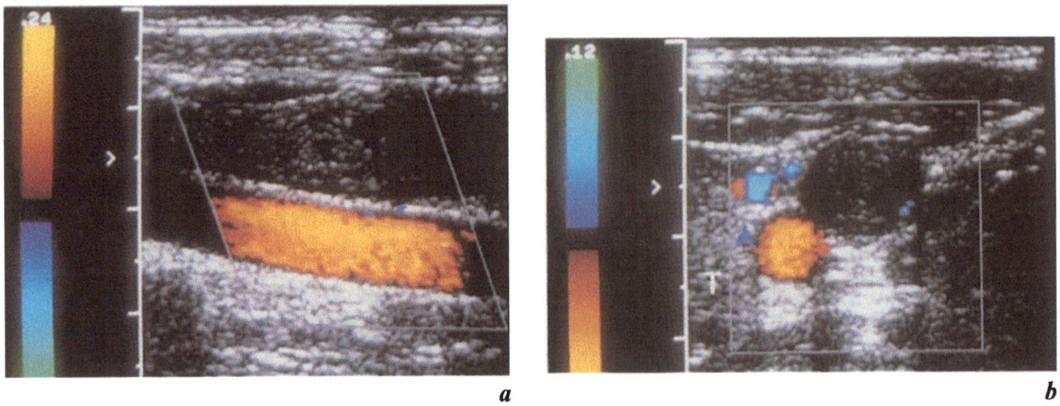

Fig. 10. Recent thrombosis of the IJV (longitudinal and transverse sections): the thrombotic material is of low echogenicity and no flow signals are shown within the vein; the common carotid artery is shown in red (T = thyroid gland)

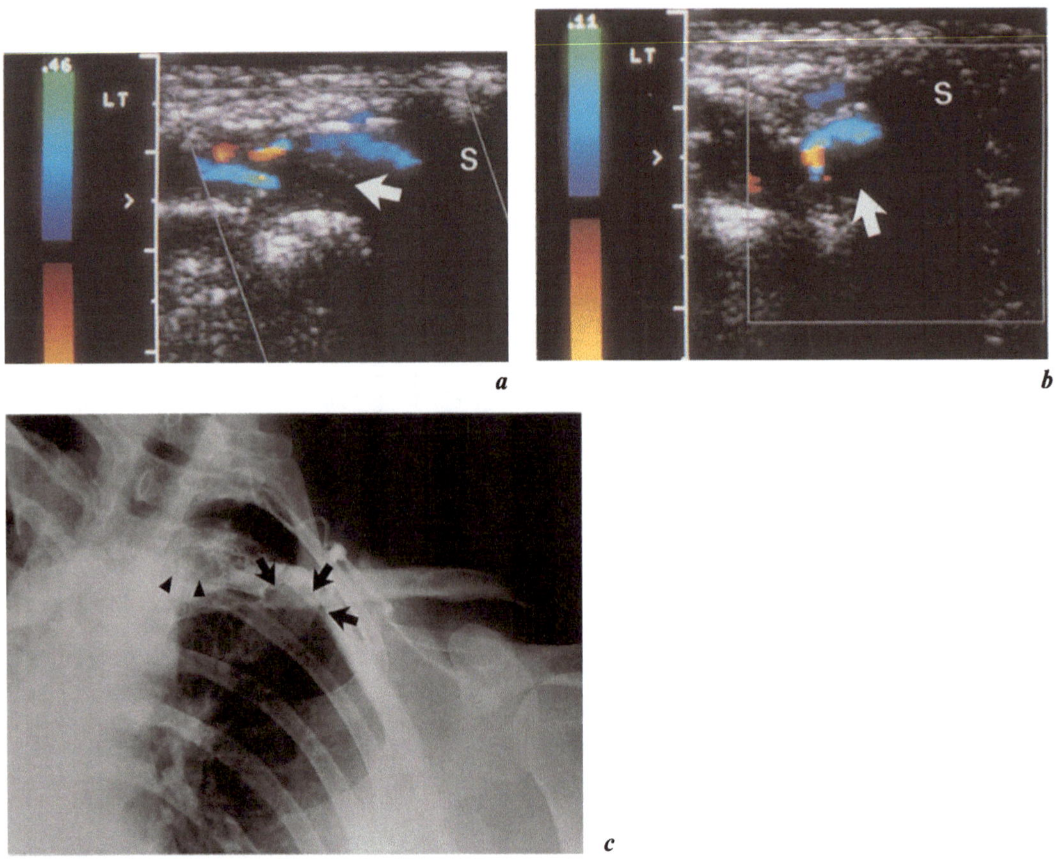

Fig. 11a. Longitudinal section of the left subclavian vein in a 25 year old female patient with pulmonary embolism confirmed by scintigraphy: the medial aspect of the subclavian vein in this case could only be demonstrated from a supraclavicular approach (S = shadowing caused by the clavicle). The arrow indicates an area devoid of color display of blood flow corresponding to an area of thrombus along the vessel wall; thrombosis of the vein is not complete, however

Fig. 11b. Transverse section of the same site illustrated in Fig. 11a: the presence of a thrombus (arrow) adherent to the vessel wall is confirmed (S = shadowing by the clavicle)

Fig. 11c. Same patient as Fig. 11a/b: venography shows a filling defect at the same location (arrows); small collaterals are visible and there is an inflow phenomenon caused by the IJV (arrowheads); the brachiocephalic vein appears normal

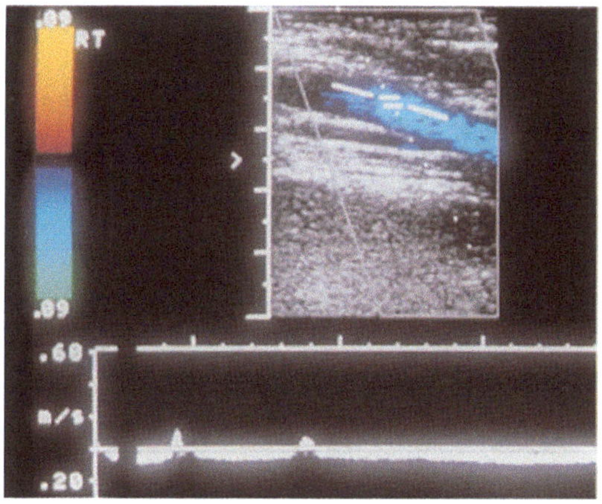

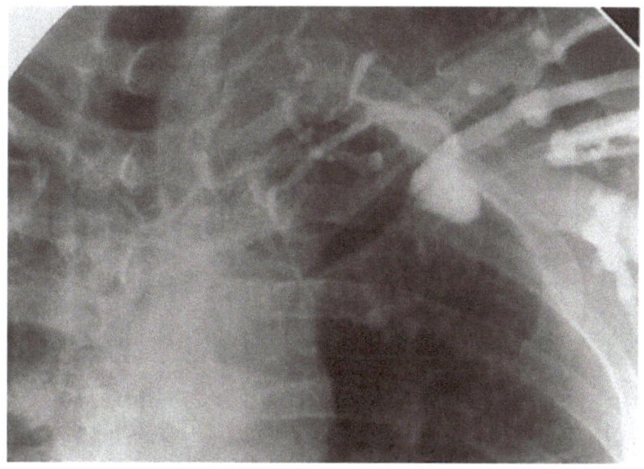

a *b*

Fig. 12a. CCDS of the axillary/subclavian vein reveals lack of cyclic change of blood flow velocity as well as low velocity of blood flow; these findings are consistent with thrombosis of the brachiocephalic vein

Fig. 12b. Venography of the subclavian vein (same patient as shown in Fig. 12a): thrombosis of the brachiocephalic vein and a portion of the subclavian vein is confirmed; moderate collateralization is present. Thrombosis of the IJV was also demonstrated by CCDS in this patient

Table 1. Diagnostic criteria for venous thrombosis

– Intraluminal echogenic material (homogenous or inhomogenous)
– Loss of compressibility of the vein
– No augmentation during Valsalva maneuver
– Absence of flow signals in duplex Doppler sonography or CCDS in the entire vessel or parts of the vessel

Thrombosis of the brachiocephalic veins cannot be assessed directly, but indirect evidence may include reduced flow in the ipsilateral subclavian and internal jugular veins as compared to the contralateral vessels and loss of normal cyclic changes in flow velocity (Fig. 12a, b). These changes are not pathognomonic of brachiocephalic vein thrombosis since similar findings may be present when there is compromised venous flow due to vein narrowing or compression, as in the presence of a mediastinal mass. False negative results may also occur when CCDS is used for evaluation of central venous thrombosis; a study of 22 patients with imaging correlation showed a sensitivity of only 78% but a high specificity of 90% for CCDS.

CCDS is better than duplex Doppler sonography in the detection of minimal flow in cases of incomplete thrombosis or early recanalization after thrombolytic therapy (Fig. 14). CCDS may also help in the demonstration of the formation of venous collateral channels; one setting in which this can be seen occurs when thrombus emerging from the subclavian vein causes occlusion of the caudad portion of the internal jugular vein: the more cephalad portion of the IJV often remains patent because of available collateral pathways via the superior thyroidal veins (Fig. 13).

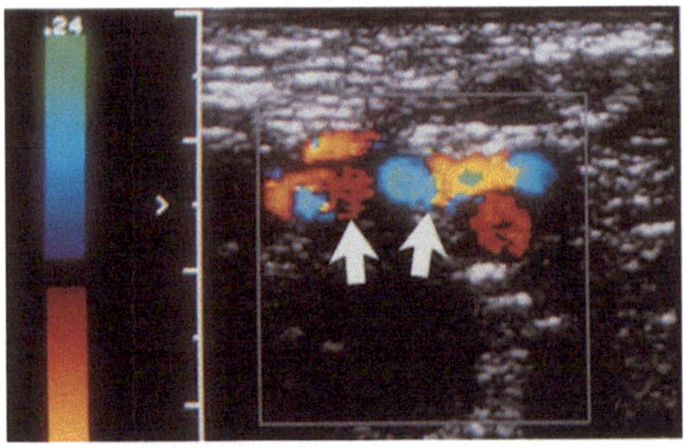

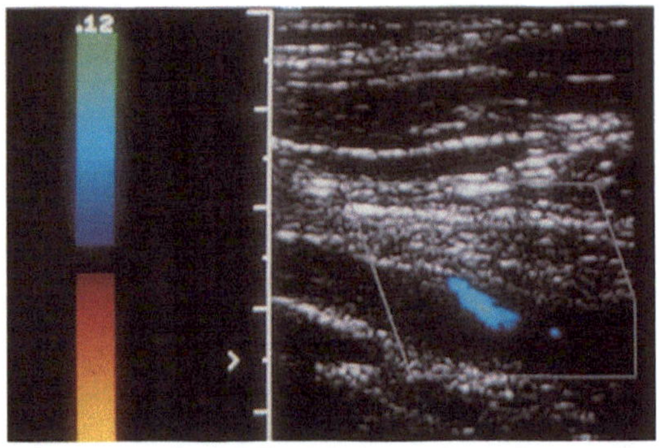

Fig. 13. (left) Transverse section at the level of the superior pole of the thyroid gland (left side): collateral drainage via the superior thyroidal veins (arrows) is present in this patient with thrombosis of the inferior part of the IJV (common carotid artery shown in red)

Fig. 14. (right) Recanalization of the subclavian vein during anticoagulation with Phenprocoumon: the thin string of color indicates beginning recanalization; the remainder of the vessel lumen is filled by thrombotic material of low echogenicity

2. Venous abnormalities related to malignant disease

The deep cervical lymph nodes are located along the internal jugular vein. Because of this close anatomic relationship enlarged lymph nodes from metastatic malignant disease may cause displacement or compression of the vein, usually from the ventral aspect (Figs. 15, 16). The IJV can also be affected by primary tumors such as large carcinomas of the tongue or tonsils or anaplastic carcinoma of the thyroid gland.

The subclavian and axillary veins are also accompanied by lymph nodes which, when enlarged, can lead to compromised vessel function (Fig. 17). In some cases, metastatic lymph nodes may have very low echogenicity; CCDS is helpful in correctly identifying the vessel lumen and demonstrating areas of intimate contact of metastatic lymph nodes or primary tumor with the arteries and veins. This

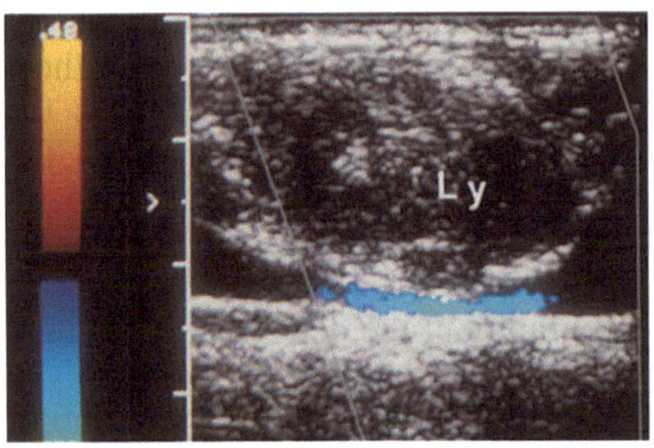

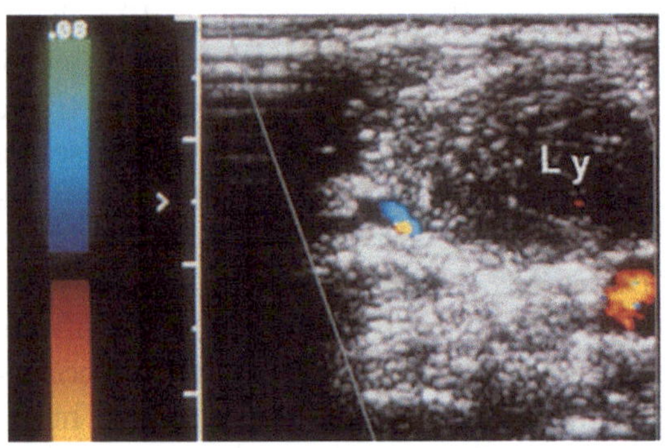

Fig. 15. (left) Compression of the IJV (longitudinal section) by a lymph node enlarged by metastatic tumor. An enlarged lymph node with inhomogenous structure (Ly) is visualized ventral to the vein which is patent but markedly narrowed

Fig. 16. (right) Same case as Fig. 15: the enlarged lymph node (Ly) not only causes IJV compression but also displaces it from its normal course (blue: IJV; red: common carotid artery)

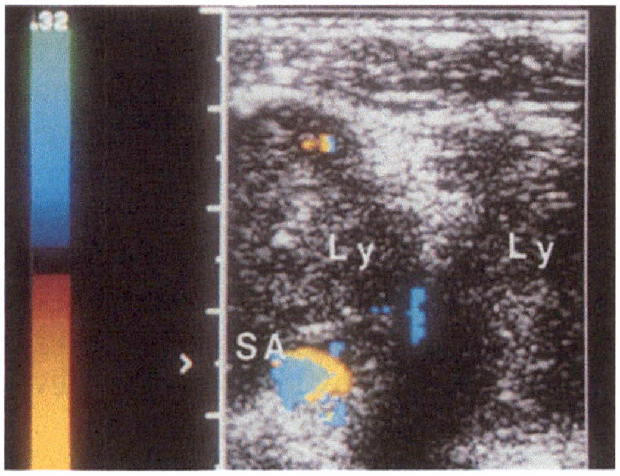

Fig. 17. Transverse section of subclavian artery and vein: enlarged lymph nodes (Ly) are shown surrounding the vessels in this patient with a melanoma of the back; note the intimate contact between the enlarged nodes and subclavian vein (blue) as well as obvious venous compression (SA = subclavian artery)

important information can be provided preoperatively to the surgeon who may then make a better assessment of the likelihood of malignant infiltration of vessel walls. This becomes especially critical in cases of bilateral metastases; if at least one side can be shown to lack involvement of the internal jugular vein then it is possible to preserve venous flow at least unilaterally. This will spare the patient the increased risk of severe head and neck edema and those cerebral complications known to be associated with simultaneous bilateral ligation or resection of the internal jugular veins.

3. Postoperative findings

In radical neck dissection, the IJV is resected; postoperative scans will often demonstrate a "stump" representing the inferior bulb in the lower part of the neck. Where tumor spread necessitates bilateral radical neck dissection the problems mentioned above (severe head and neck edema and potential cerebral complications) have led to the development of several methods of venous reconstruction. CCDS is useful in postoperative evaluation of the success of these procedures.

4. Anomalies

Anomalies of the IJV are rare. The vein is never completely absent, but sometimes it is very small. A rare variant is duplication of the IJV; the two venous channels usually communicate at their cranial and caudal ends. Congenital phlebectasia of the IJV presents clinically as a swelling in the neck which enlarges during the Valsalva maneuver; this condition can readily be differentiated from a cervical cyst by CCDS or duplex Doppler sonography.

Conclusion

Imaging procedures are indispensable for the diagnosis of thrombosis of the internal jugular and subclavian veins. CCDS has proven to be a suitable alternative to venography, especially in the assessment of the internal jugular vein for thrombosis (where venography, CT, or MRI are now needed only when there is special concern about the region of the superior bulb or brachiocephalic veins). In malignant disease, compression or displacement of the veins by enlarged lymph nodes is better assessed by sonography than by venography. Although venous thrombosis or other entities can also be diagnosed by duplex Doppler sonography and sometimes even by B-mode imaging, CCDS makes the process more rapid and accurate.

References

Adams JT, McEvoy RK, DeWeese JA (1965) Primary deep venous thrombosis of upper extremity. Arch Surg 91:29–35

Brownlow Jr RL, McKinney WM (1985) Ultrasonic evaluation of jugular venous valve competence. J Ultrasound Med 4:169–172

Campbell CB, Chandler JG, Tegtmeyer CJ (1977) Axillary, subclavian and brachiocephalic obstruction. Surgery 82:816–822

Comerota AJ, Harwick RD, White JV (1986) Jugular venous reconstruction: A technique to minimize morbidity of bilateral radical neck dissection. J Vasc Surg 3:322–329

Dresser LP, McKinney WM (1987) Anatomic and pathophysiologic studies of the human internal jugular valve. Am J Surgery 154:220–224

Fitzgerald SP, Leckie WJH (1985) Thrombosis complicating transvenous pacemaker lead presenting as contralateral IJV occlusion. Am Heart J 109:593–595

Grassi JC, Polak JF (1990) Axillary and subclavian venous thrombosis: Follow-up evaluation with color Doppler flow US and venography. Radiology 175:651–654

Gritzmann N, Grasl MCh, Helmer M, Steiner E (1990) Invasion of the carotid artery and jugular vein by lymph node metastases: Detection with sonography. AJR 154:411–414

Gritzmann N, Czembirek H, Hajek P, Karnel F, Frühwald F (1987) Sonographische Halsanatomie und ihre Bedeutung beim Lymphknotenstaging von Kopf-Hals-Malignomen. Fortschr Röntgenstr 146:1–7

Falk RL, Smith DF (1987) Thrombosis of upper extremity thoracic inlet veins: Diagnosis with duplex Doppler sonography. AJR 149:677–682

Gaitini D, Kaftori JK, Pery M, Engel A (1988) High resolution real-time ultrasonography: Diagnosis and follow-up of jugular and subclavian vein thrombosis. J Ultrasound Med 7:621–627

Gooding GAW, Hightower DR, Moore DH, Dillon WP, Lipton MJ (1986) Obstruction of the superior vena cava or subclavian veins: Sonographic diagnosis. Radiology 159:663–665

Huber P, Häuptli W, Schmitt HE (1987) Die Axillar-Subclaviathrombose and ihre Folgen. Internist 28:336–342

Hübsch PJS, Stiglbauer RL, Schwaighofer BW, Kainberger FM, Barton PP (1988) Internal jugular and subclavian vein thrombosis caused by central venous catheters. Evaluation using Doppler blood flow imaging. J Ultrasound Med 7:629–636

Hedtler W, Geissmann A, Berchtold C (1987) Sonographie bei Jugularvenenthrombose. Ultraschall 8:237–238

Hightower DR, Gooding GAW (1985) Sonographic evaluation of the normal response of subclavian veins to respiratory maneuvers. Invest Radiol 20:517–520

Jost U (1983) Massive Thrombose durch Shaldon-Katheter zur Langzeit-Hämodialyse and Plasmapherese über die Vena jugularis interna. Anaesthesist 32:560–562

Kerr TM, Lutter KS, Moeller DM, Hasselfeld KA, Roedersheimer LR, McKenna PJ, Winkler JL, Spirtoff K, Sampson MG, Cranley JJ (1990) Upper extremity venous thrombosis diagnosed by duplex scanning. Am J Surg 160:202–206

Knudson GJ, Wiedmeyer DA, Erickson SJ, Foley WD, Lawson TL, Mewissen MW, Lipchik EO (1990) Color Doppler sonographic imaging in the assessment of upper-extremity deep venous thrombosis. AJR 154:399–403

König R, Mukhopadhyay CH, Gademann G, Lorenz D (1986) Sonographischer, computertomographischer und kernspintomographischer Nachweis einer Thrombose der V. jugularis interna. Fortschr Röntgenstr 144:611–614

von Lanz T, Wachsmuth W (1955) Praktische Anatomie, Bd I, 2. Teil: Hals. Springer, Berlin Göttingen Heidelberg

Leung A, Hampson SJ, Singh MP, Charr D (1983) Ultrasonic diagnosis of bilateral congenital jugular venous aneurysms. Br J Rad 56:588–591

Schmidt RF, Thews G (Hrsg) (1980) Physiologie des Menschen, 20. Aufl. Springer, Berlin Heidelberg New York

Terwey B, Krier C, Gerhardt P (1981) Die Darstellung der Jugularvenenthrombose mit Hilfe des hochauflösenden Ultraschallverfahrens. Fortschr Röntgenstr 134:557–559

Tilney NL, Griffiths HJ, Edwards EA (1970) Natural history of major venous thrombosis of the upper extremity. Arch Surg 101:792–796

Wing V, Scheible W (1983) Sonography of jugular vein thrombosis. AJR 140:333–336

Warwick R, Williams PL (eds) (1989) Gray's anatomy, 37th edn. Churchill Livingstone, Edinburgh London Melbourne New York

Yiengpruksawan A, Ganepola GA, Freeman HP (1987) Thrombosis of noncatheterized internal jugular vein: A unique complication of subclavian catheterization diagnosed by ultrasound. J Natl Med Assoc 79:961–965

Yokomori K, Kubo K, Kanamori Y, Takemura T, Yamamoto T (1990) Internal jugular phlebectasia in two siblings: manometric and histopathologic studies of the pathogenesis. J Pediatr Surg 25:762–765

Zanella FE, Brusis T, Moedder U (1986) Der Einsatz bildgebender Verfahren in der Diagnostik der Jugularvenenthrombose. Laryngol Rhinol Otol 65:322–326

Zohar Y, Ben-Tovim R, Talmi YP (1989) Phlebectasia of the jugular system. J Craniomaxillofac Surg 17:96–98

8
Color-coded Doppler sonography of dialysis fistulas

P. Hübsch and S. Trattnig

Introduction

Current therapeutic options for the treatment of chronic uremia require a multidisciplinary approach in which nephrologists, urologists and other surgeons, and radiologists must work together to achieve maximum benefit for the patient. Because of the interventional techniques now available, the radiologist has a very active role to play in the treatment of malfunctioning dialysis fistulas. The main purpose of this chapter is to describe the potential diagnostic value of color-coded Doppler sonography (CCDS) in the noninvasive evaluation of hemodialysis fistulas. It should be noted that angiography (preferably digital subtraction angiography) still holds its position as a "gold standard" shunt evaluation method and can provide more accurate and complete information than CCDS. The two procedures probably have a complementary role to play, as is often the case when new medical diagnostic modalities become available. In the following sections we will discuss the typical appearance of pathologic changes occurring in dialysis fistulas and will also note the difficulties which can be encountered when using CCDS in the diagnostic work-up of patients with shunt malfunction.

General principles

A prerequisite for long-term hemodialysis treatment in uremic patients is some method of ready vascular access. In an acute setting a central venous catheter (such as a Shaldon catheter, Permcath (Quinton) catheter, etc.) can be used, most commonly by way of the internal jugular vein or subclavian vein. This type of catheter cannot, however, be used for more than a short period of time; if hemodialysis is to be continued on a long-term basis another type of access must be provided. Surgical arteriovenous fistulas are created to provide the patient with a vessel which can be easily punctured with a 15 or 16-gauge needle and which is capable of providing adequate blood flow (at least 150–300 ml/min). The procedure of choice today is formation of such a fistula in the forearm (introduced by Brescia and Cimino in 1966); this has largely replaced the use of such extracorporeal systems as the Scribner shunt which has been available for several decades.

The forearm fistula consists of an anastomosis between the radial artery and the cephalic vein (Fig. 1); less often, the ulnar artery is used in the creation of the fistula. Since almost all fistulas eventually become unsuitable for use in dialysis they are initially placed as distally as possible; this allows the surgeon to create new fistulas at more proximal levels when needed. The non-dominant arm is used whenever possible.

Approaches currently in use besides the Brescia-Cimino fistula include placement of synthetic grafts made of polytetrafluoroethylene (PTFE, Gore-Tex™), generally in a U-shaped manner (Fig. 2). The graft then serves as a connection between an artery and a vein. Cadaver veins or bovine heterografts (carotid arteries) are only occasionally used for this purpose.

Meticulous operative technique and careful management of the fistula help to keep the complication rate low. Nevertheless, the patency rate 12 months after surgery is only 65–85% depending on the type of the shunt. Proper puncture technique is of critical importance in maximizing the useful life of a shunt. In the case of the Brescia-Cimino fistula this involves use of the *venous* portion of the fistula, where one needle is placed distally for the extraction of blood and a second needle is placed proximally for returning dialyzed blood to the patient's circulation.

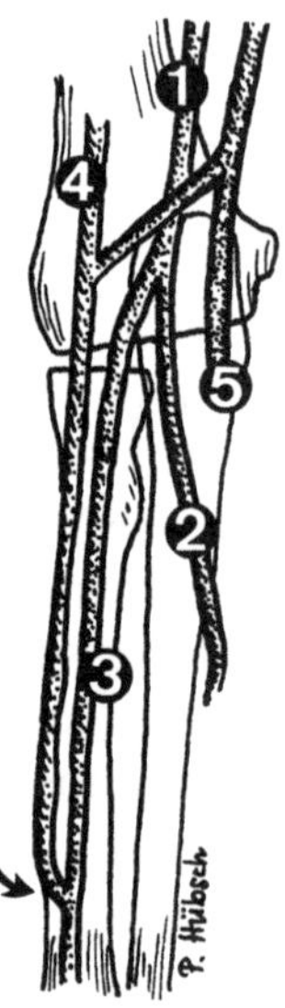

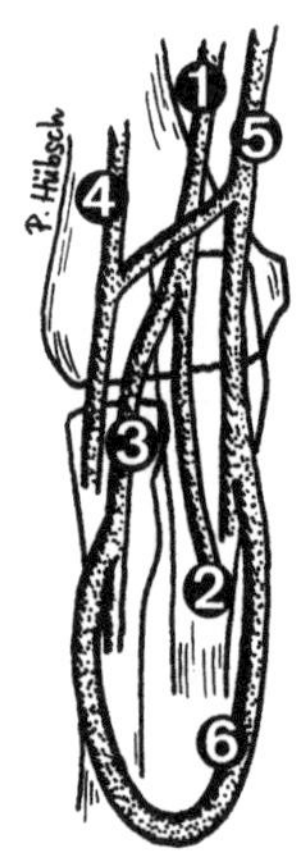

Fig. 1. (left) Brescia-Cimino dialysis fistula in the forearm: (1) brachial artery (2) ulnar artery (3) radial artery (4) cephalic vein (5) basilic vein. The anastomosis is indicated by an arrow

Fig. 2. (right) Example of a polytetrafluoroethylene (PTFE) graft: (1) brachial artery (2) ulnar artery (3) radial artery (4) cephalic vein (5) basilic vein (6) graft

The repeated trauma to this segment of the fistula can lead to complications, so careful assessment of this area as well as the sites of surgical anastomoses should be carried out when using imaging techniques.

Examination technique

The sonographic examination of dialysis fistulas should not be limited to the anastomosis and the adjacent vein (although these are the regions where most of the problems occur), but must include all vessels which are sonographically visible and are of importance for the maintenance of an adequate flow rate across the shunt. This means that the subclavian artery, the brachial artery, the radial and ulnar arteries, the anastomosis, and the venous outflow tract up to the subclavian vein must be examined. A Doppler spectral tracing should be obtained at least from the artery proximal to the anastomosis, the anastomosis itself, and the adjacent vein. It is useful to employ pulsed Doppler with angle correction as often as possible in addition to CCDS for documentation of absolute blood flow velocity and the relationship between systolic and diastolic velocity. To quantify this relationship the resistive index (see "Examination Technique" section of vertebral artery chapter) can be calculated. The calculation of the shunt volume (in ml/min) on the basis of mean flow velocity and the diameter of the vessel seems to be unnecessary in all but selected cases; this is due to two factors: the flow volume calculations are not always accurate, and dialysis pressure is a good indicator of shunt dysfunction.

All vessels should be examined in longitudinal and transverse planes: Table 1 outlines our protocol for evaluation of a fistula of the Brescia-Cimino type. This approach is applicable to other types of fistulas with only minor modifications.

Table 1. Protocol for CCDS of a dialysis fistula of the Brescia-Cimino type

1. Examination of the arterial limb, including subclavian, axillary and brachial artery in longitudinal sections, moving from the subclavian artery distally.
2. Examination of the anastomosis in longitudinal and transverse sections.
3. Tracing of artery and vein proximally in transverse planes.
4. Examination of the veins up to the subclavian vein in longitudinal sections.

In addition to the above-mentioned principles and some general assumptions such as the availability of a linear scanhead with a frequency of at least 5 MHz (or even better, 7 MHz or greater), there are some other points which should be emphasized. Since any irregularity of the vessel wall may lead to future complications, especially thrombus formation, it is important to search carefully for such "intimal flaps". If CCDS alone is used for vessel evaluation the superimposed color may obscure small areas of wall irregularity. It is therefore important to use B-mode technique alone for vessel wall demonstration, especially in the venous limb of the fistula which, as noted above, is subject to repeated intimal trauma from needle punctures (Fig. 3).

Scan technique is another important factor. Excessive pressure applied by the scanhead can cause alterations in morphological appearance of the anastomosis and the venous limb of the fistula and can alter local blood flow characteristics.

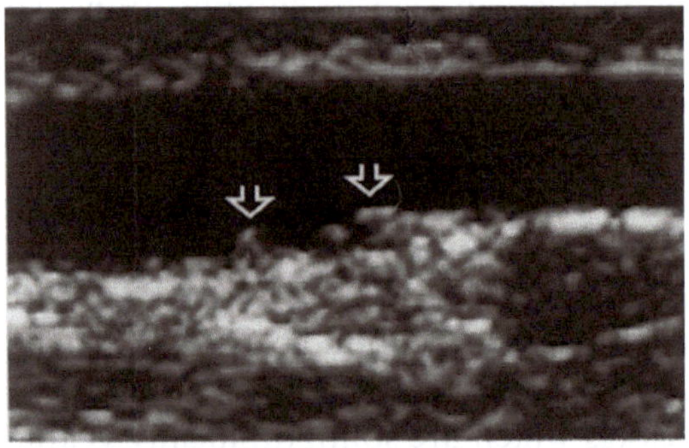

Fig. 3. Irregularities of the vessel wall (arrows) in the venous limb of a dialysis fistula. These "intimal flaps" may be better demonstrated by conventional B-mode ultrasound since they are sometimes obscured by overlaid color when CCDS is used

Proper technique involves the generous use of scanning gel and use of only enough pressure to maintain consistent transmission of sound.

The sensitivity of the color Doppler unit has to be adjusted individually for each arterial, venous, or anastomotic site evaluated in order to compensate for variations in blood flow velocity and any color artifacts encountered. One commonly encountered artifact occurs when vibrations in the perivascular soft tissues lead to color-encoding of extraluminal portions of the image. This is most commonly noted near the anastomosis and venous limb of the fistula (Fig. 4); it can be present even when the anastomosis is functioning normally but can also be caused by increased turbulence related to stenosis. This type of artifact can often be minimized or eliminated by careful adjustment of sensitivity of the color display, or by moderate manual compression of the feeding artery. If these measures are not successful then duplex Doppler sonography without color display should be utilized so that a vascular lesion is not overlooked or a false-positive impression of stenosis obtained.

Artifacts can also arise within the vessel lumen due to aliasing in areas of high-velocity flow; this can be difficult to distinguish from turbulence (see carotid artery chapter). Aliasing can be minimized to some extent by reduction of color

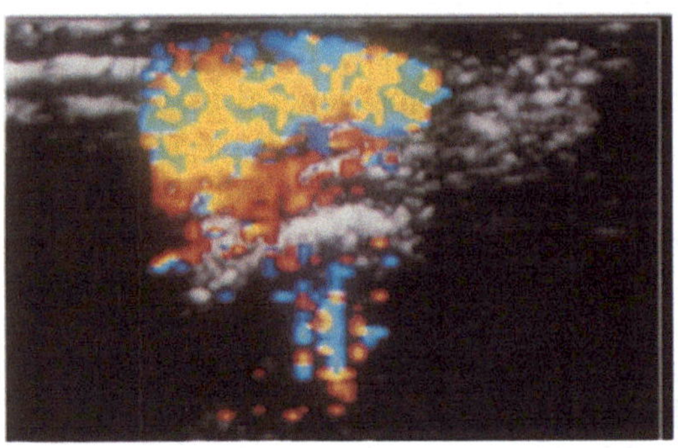

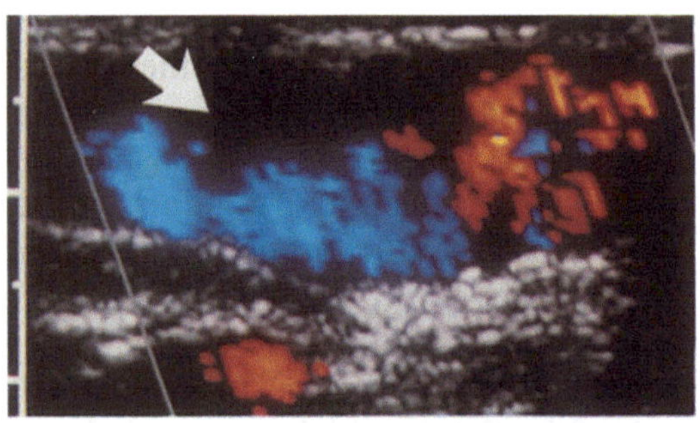

Fig. 4. (left) Extensive perivascular color artifacts around the anastomosis in a Brescia-Cimino fistula due to incorrect sensitivity adjustment of color display; the vessel is not adequately visualized

Fig. 5. (right) Reduction of the sensitivity of the CCDS unit for the detection of motion may produce areas with no color display near the vessel wall (arrow). This must not be confused with vessel wall thrombus

display sensitivity, but this may cause complete loss of color-coding where flow velocity is lowest, mainly along the vessel wall (Fig. 5); such areas must not be mistaken for thrombus formation.

Normal CCDS appearance of dialysis fistulas

The artery supplying the fistula is characterized by high flow velocities in both systole and diastole, resulting in a low resistive index; this is the expected in finding the presence of low peripheral resistance typical of an arteriovenous shunt of any kind. Absolute velocities during systole and diastole are variable and depend on cardiac output as well as on the shunt volume. Broadening of the Doppler spectrum in pulsed Doppler examination indicating slightly turbulent flow may occur but is not always present (Fig. 6). At the site of the anastomosis, which usually runs in a transverse direction with respect to the ulna and radius (Figs. 7, 8), the blood flow is usually turbulent; CCDS images will show a characteristic varicolored pattern, and concurrent recording of the pulsed Doppler waveform will show spectral broadening. Sometimes a Doppler waveform with signals above and below the zero line with irregular amplitude can be recorded, which closely resembles the pattern from arteriovenous fistulas at other sites in the body.

Similarly, signs of turbulent flow can be observed in the venous limb of the dialysis fistula (Fig. 9). Both CCDS and conventional Doppler waveform tracings show decreasing evidence of turbulence with increasing distance from the anasto-

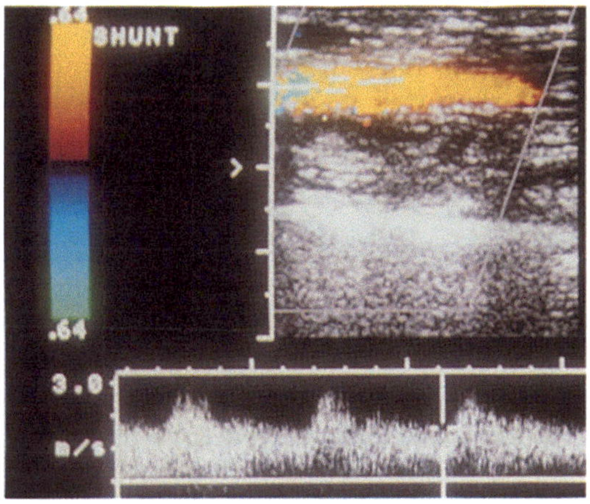

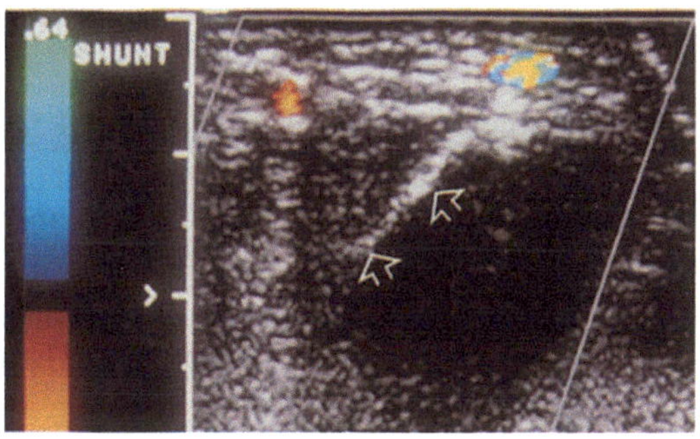

Fig. 6. (left) Normal arterial limb of a dialysis fistula: CCDS shows color in the vessel lumen during systole and diastole with no reversed component of blood flow during diastole. The spectral waveform is typical of an A-V communication, with high diastolic blood flow velocity due to low peripheral resistance. Slight broadening of the Doppler spectrum indicates some turbulence (this finding may or may not be present in a normal fistula)

Fig. 7. (right) Transverse section immediately proximal to the anastomosis between radial artery (red) and cephalic vein in a normal dialysis fistula of the Brescia-Cimino type. The surface of the radius produces a thin echogenic line with shadowing (arrows)

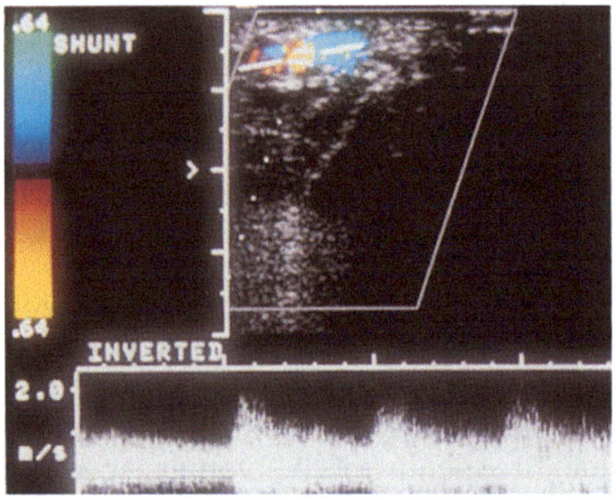

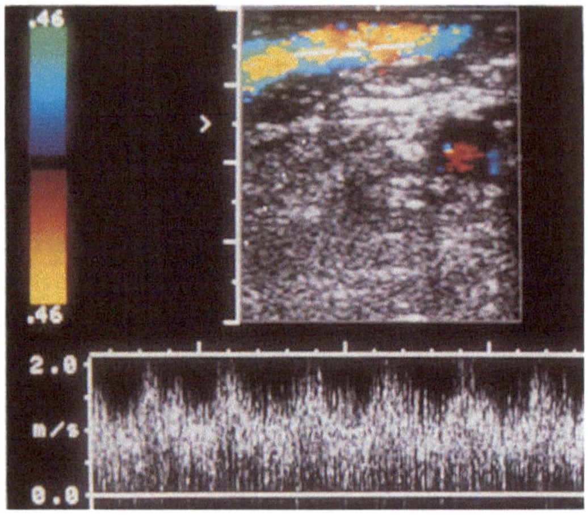

Fig. 8. (left) Typical appearance of an anastomosis; the Doppler waveform shows spectral broadening (filling in of the area under the wave outline due to many different frequency components occurring simultaneously because of turbulence)

Fig. 9. (right) Normal venous limb (distal part) close to the anastomosis in a dialysis fistula: the typical varicolored picture and the broadening shown on the spectral waveform tracing indicate marked turbulence; aliasing artifacts also can occur. The Doppler waveform also shows a systolic increase similar to an arterial pattern

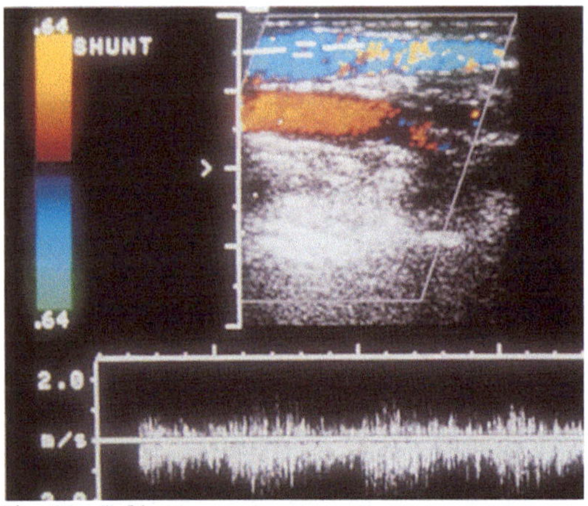

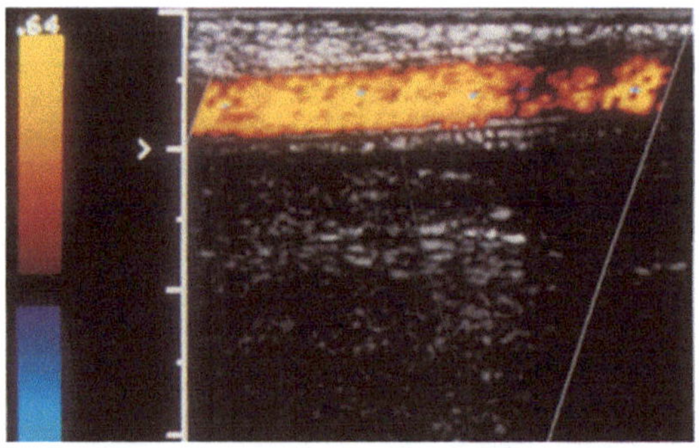

Fig. 10. (left) Normal venous limb (proximal part) further from the anastomosis in a dialysis fistula: the systolic velocity peaks are less prominent than in the distal part reflecting increased distance from the feeding artery. The Doppler spectrum shows varying amplitudes

Fig. 11. (right) Typical appearance of a polytetrafluoroethylene (PTFE) graft: the wall of the graft is represented by two thin echogenic lines. There is marked sound attenuation deep to the graft

mosis. The systolic peaks, reflective of arterial-type flow in the vein near the anastomosis, also become less prominent as sampling is carried out further and further from the anastomotic site (Fig. 10).

PTFE grafts present with a clearly definable wall and sound attenuation deep to the graft (Fig. 11) which allows precise identification of the anastomotic sites.

Pathologic findings

1. Stenosis

Stenosis in any part of the dialysis fistula (feeding artery, anastomosis, or venous outflow tract) carries with it the threat of loss of the site for vascular access since thrombosis is likely to occur. It is for this reason that early detection is essential so that percutaneous transluminal angioplasty (PTA) can be carried out for both short- and long-term salvage of the fistula. About 50–70% of the stenoses occur in the venous limb of the fistula near the anastomosis. Another 20% are found at the anastomotic site, and the feeding artery is the site of stenosis in no more than 10% of cases. The rest of the stenoses occur in the proximal and central veins (proximal cephalic vein, subclavian vein, and brachiocephalic vein). In a series of patients undergoing angiography because of a malfunctioning dialysis fistula, central venous stenosis was found in as many as 14%. In some cases this may be related to previous insertion of central venous catheters, but more often the cause for such a high incidence of central venous stenosis remains uncertain.

Figures 12–15 show examples of stenoses at different sites with angiographic correlation. The criteria for stenosis are the same as for the arterial system in general: visible narrowing of the vessel lumen, marked increase in blood flow velocity relative to the pre-stenotic portion of the vessel, and turbulence; as the degree of stenosis becomes increasingly severe a point will be reached where velocity increase is no longer present. CCDS is reported to detect stenosis with a sensitivity of about 90%. Most of the stenoses that are missed by CCDS are located in the proximal or central veins. Reversed flow direction in the internal jugular vein or low flow velocity in the subclavian vein during inspiration may indicate high-grade stenosis of the brachiocephalic vein (which is not visible sonographically because of overlying bone).

As mentioned above, vascular stenosis (especially when located at or near the anastomosis) may cause perivascular tissue vibration and resultant color artifacts (Fig. 16). The presence of such artifactual color changes is not, however, patho-

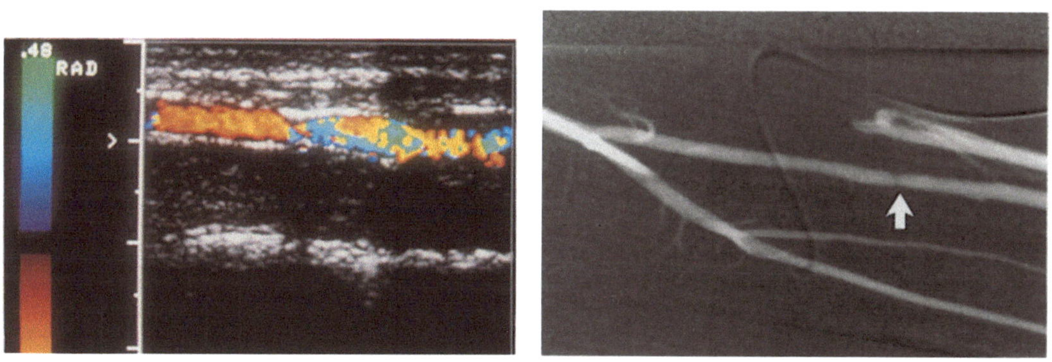

a *b*

Fig. 12a. Stenosis of the radial artery proximal to the anastomosis: post-stenotic turbulence (varicolored appearance) is evident in the CCDS image; lighter colors indicate moderate blood flow acceleration

Fig. 12b. Angiographic confirmation (early arterial phase) of the CCDS findings shown in Fig. 12a: moderate stenosis in the proximal part of the radial artery is present (arrow)

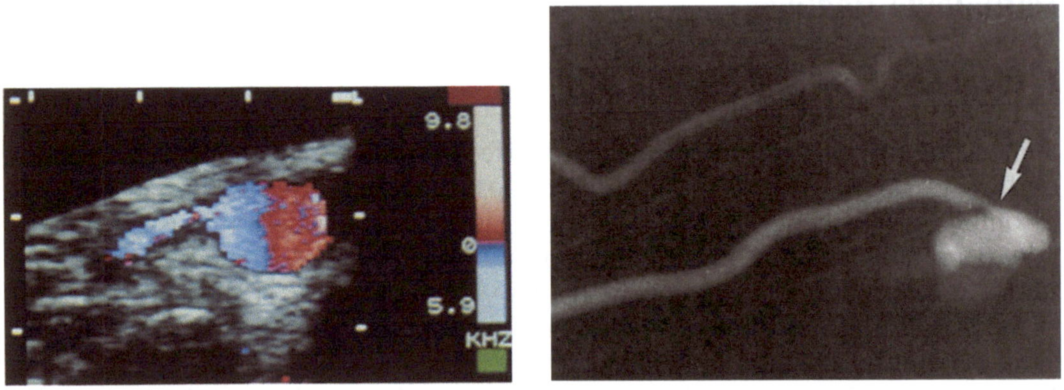

a b

Fig. 13a. CCDS of the anastomosis in a Brescia-Cimino fistula: there is marked narrowing of the vessel lumen, which is outlined by color

Fig. 13b. Angiographic confirmation (early arterial phase) of the CCDS finding shown in Fig. 13a: there is a short, tight stenosis (arrow) in the region of the anastomosis (an aneurysm is also present adjacent to the stenosis)

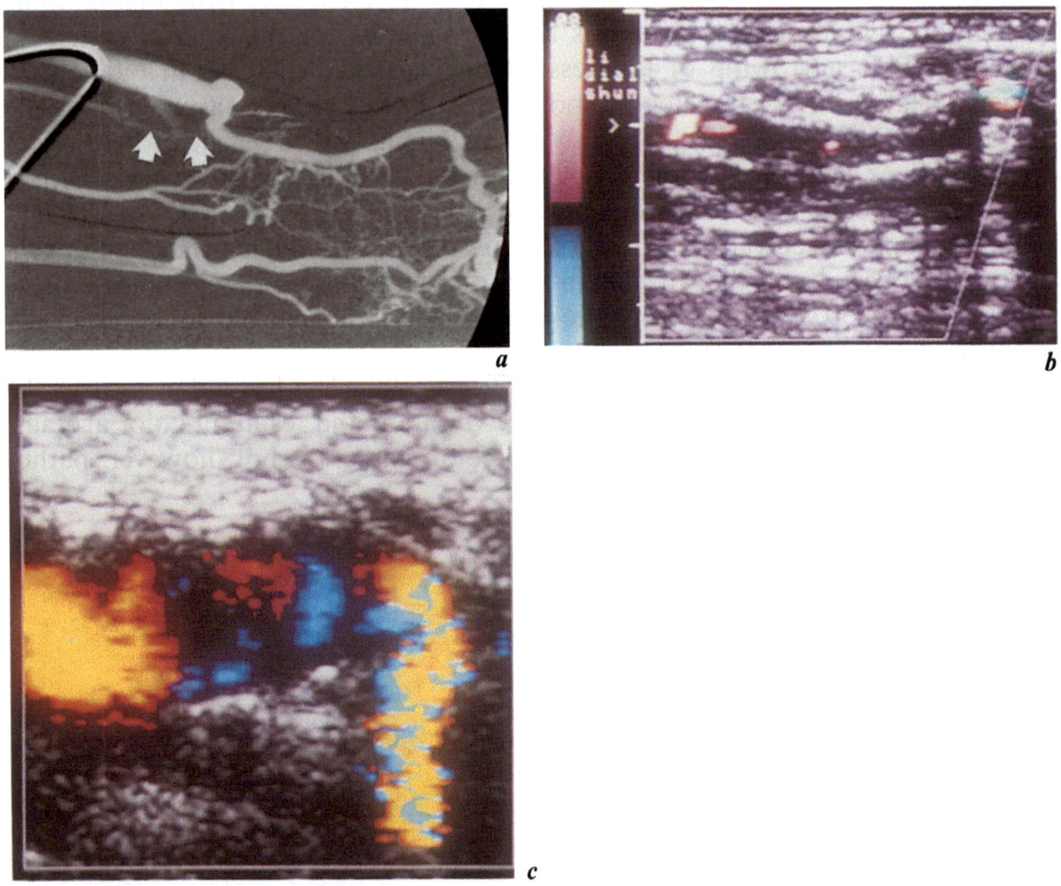

a b c

Fig. 14a. The angiogram shows a subtotal stenosis of the radial artery proximal to the anastomosis, with only minimal filling of the vessel (arrows). The anastomosis itself appears normal; there is collateralization through the deep palmar arch with good venous runoff

Fig. 14b. CCDS clearly demonstrates the subtotal stenosis of the radial artery indicated by arrows in Fig. 14a. Only minimal flow is demonstrated (red dots along lumen)

Fig. 14c. The retrograde filling of the anastomosis (see Fig. 14a) is readily demonstrated by CCDS

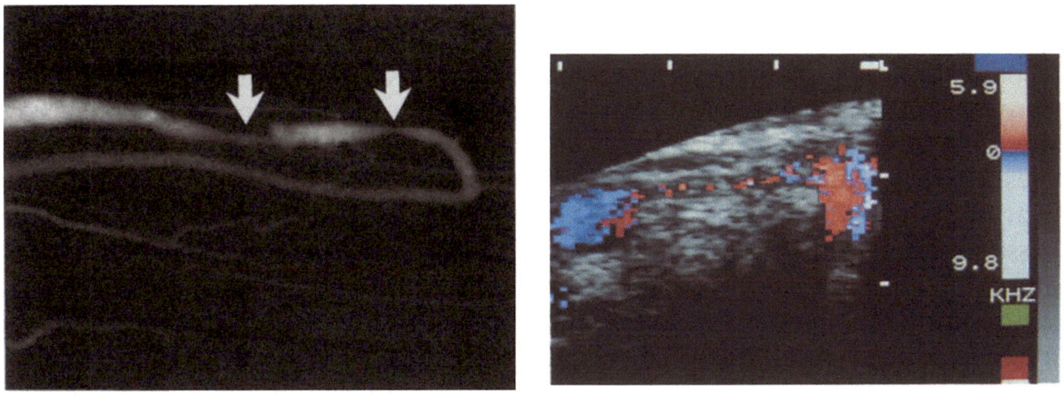

a *b*

Fig. 15a. Angiography shows two high-grade stenoses of the venous limb of the dialysis fistula (arrows)

Fig. 15b. CCDS corresponding to the angiographic findings shown in Fig. 15a demonstrates the venous stenosis

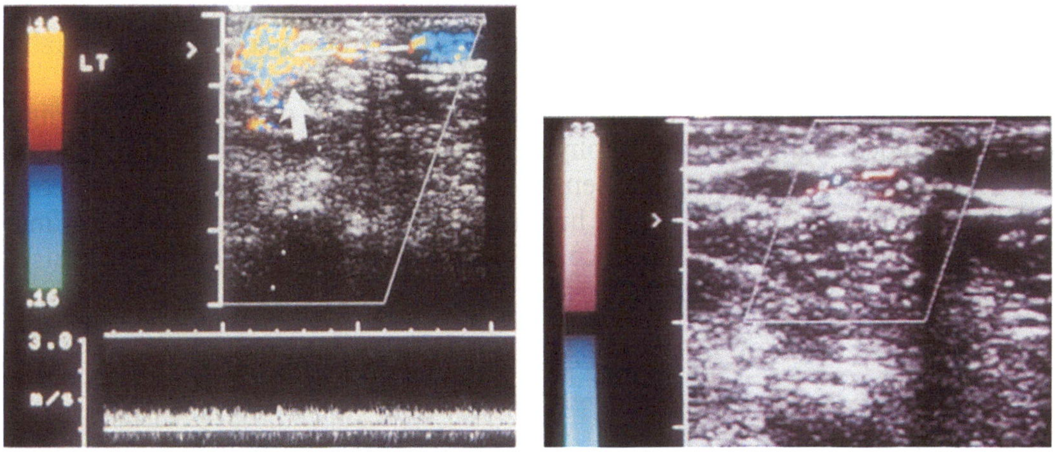

a *b*

Fig. 16a. Marked perivascular color artifacts due to a venous stenosis: the artifacts occur only in a circumscribed segment of the vessel (arrow) where they mask the underlying stenosis. Distally (right side of the picture) there are no such artifacts and the vessel lumen is displayed normally (blue). Note the absence of systolic velocity peaks in the Doppler waveform tracing

Fig. 16b. When the sensitivity of the CCDS unit is adjusted properly, the artifacts shown in Fig. 16a disappear and the narrowing of the vessel lumen can be appreciated

gnomonic of stenosis since similar findings can also be found in relationship to normal fistulas. If significant stenosis is present in the arterial limb of the fistula or in the venous limb close to the anastomosis, Doppler spectral waveform tracings obtained from the venous limb beyond the area(s) of stenosis may no longer show the systolic velocity increase reflective of direct arterial-to-venous shunting (compare normal waveform in Fig. 9 with the abnormal pattern in Fig. 16a).

2. Thrombosis

In patients with normal dialysis pressure (measured during the hemodialysis procedure) thrombosis is not very common; only 0.13 episodes per patient per year are reported for this group of patients. In contrast, patients with elevated dialysis pressure (if left untreated) will average 1.4 episodes of thrombosis per patient per year of dialysis. In about 90% of the cases, thrombosis leading to occlusion of the vessel occurs in the venous limb of the shunt. This is often due to morphological alterations of the vessel, such as stenosis. As a rule, thrombotic occlusion of the venous limb is painless. Clinical examination reveals lack of venous pulsations and absence of the typical "thrill" or bruit, but is not always conclusive; the clinical findings need to be confirmed and more detailed information obtained by the use of imaging procedures.

Thrombosis is characterized in CCDS images by a generalized or segmental loss of color coding of the vessel lumen even when low-flow detection settings of the CCDS unit are used. Since early thrombus may appear anechoic or may produce only minimal intraluminal echoes CCDS is an ideal modality for identification of recent thrombosis because it allows immediate recognition of absence of blood flow (Fig. 17). In time, intraluminal clot shows increased echodensity (Fig. 18). If there is complete thrombosis of the venous limb or of the anastomosis without formation of venous collaterals, the diastolic blood flow velocity in the feeding artery decreases to the zero level. The arterial flow pattern may remain normal in cases where venous collateral channels provide adequate drainage.

Angiography can identify occlusion but cannot reliably demonstrate the length of the occluded segment. Sonography (especially CCDS) can establish the true proximal extent of thrombus. The sensitivity of CCDS for the detection of recent occlusion of the venous limb is very high (up to 100%); false negative results may be obtained in chronic occlusion since venous collaterals may be difficult to differentiate from the regular vascular pattern.

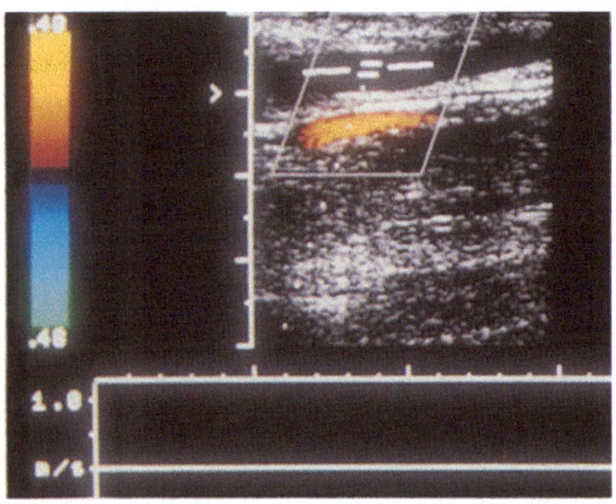

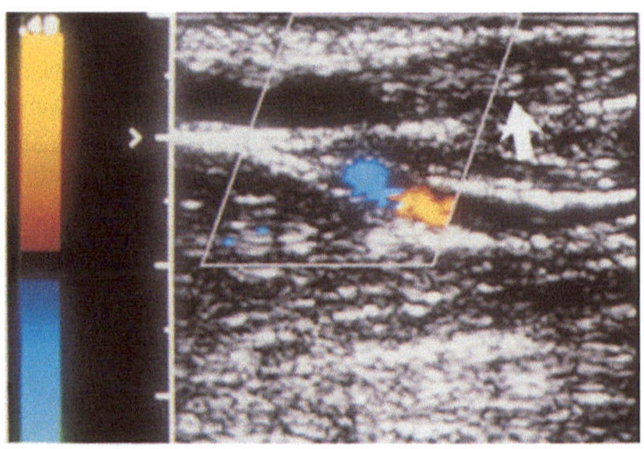

Fig. 17. (left) Recent thrombosis of the venous limb of a dialysis fistula: the vessel lumen is anechoic and no color-coding of the lumen is present; no Doppler spectrum can be recorded from the vein. Deep to the vein, the radial artery is seen (red)

Fig. 18. (right) Older thrombotic material becomes echogenic, as illustrated in this case where intraluminal clot is readily demonstrated (arrow). CCDS confirms absence of blood flow in this vein. Deep to the occluded vein a small collateral vessel is delineated by color

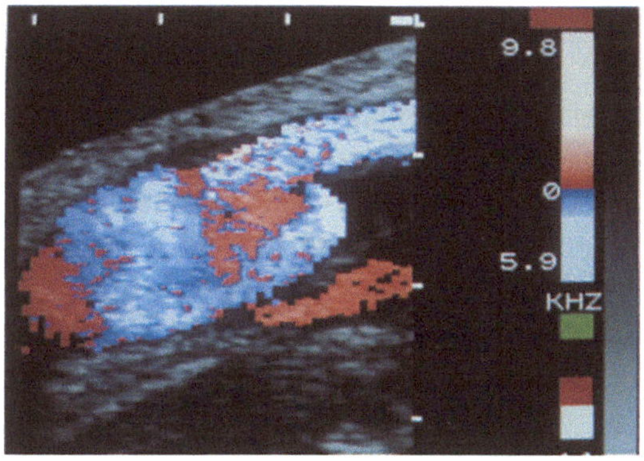

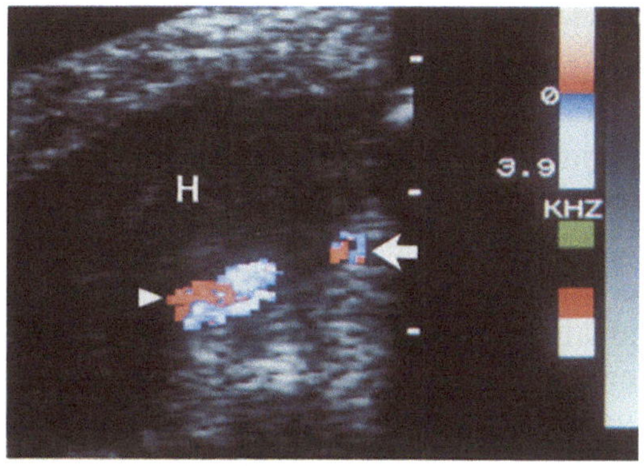

Fig. 19. (left) Typical appearance of a small aneurysm in the venous limb of a dialysis fistula

Fig. 20. (right) A recent perivascular hematoma (H) presents as a hypoechoic or anechoic area. On this transverse section, the arterial (arrow) and venous (arrowhead) limbs of the dialysis fistula are also visible next to the hematoma

3. Aneurysm

Aneurysms are almost always located in the venous limb of the dialysis fistula, perhaps as a result of exposure to arterial-type blood pressure in combination with repeated puncture trauma or by rupture of the vessel during a percutaneous transluminal angioplasty procedure. Neither angiography nor sonography can reliably differentiate true and false aneurysms; both conditions are characterized by an abrupt widening of the vessel lumen (Fig. 19). The true size of an aneurysm can be better determined by CCDS than by angiography in cases where thrombosis along the vessel wall causes narrowing of the perfused lumen. The major benefit of sonography is in rapid, noninvasive differentiation of aneurysms from perivascular hematomas. Clinical evaluation alone cannot reliably make this distinction since hematomas closely related to a vessel may show pulsations. Determination of aneurysm size is also an important role for sonography since very large aneurysms may need to be surgically excised because of the risk of rupture and severe hemorrhage.

4. Hematoma

Hematoma is a common complication of dialysis access sites; it may result from improper cannulation technique or inadequate compression after cannula removal. Fresh hematoma has a relatively low echodensity compared to the surrounding tissue (Fig. 20). The echodensity of the hematoma increases with age. Repeated large hematomas can cause limitation of access to the fistula for puncture. Sonography can help to identify an optimal site for puncture in such cases; conventional B-mode ultrasound is often adequate for this purpose.

5. Abscess

Infection leading to abscess formation is a serious complication; fortunately it is encountered only rarely. Sonography is useful for identification of liquified areas when incision and drainage is being considered. Since abscess and hematoma can have very similar sonographic morphology, clinical and laboratory findings must be taken into consideration in differential diagnosis. There can be considerable variation in echogenicity of abscesses; in those cases which show increased echodensity, "palpation" with the scanhead may cause movement of echoes within the purulent material. This should help to distinguish pus from organized blood clot since the latter tends to move as a "block" when compressed.

6. Steal syndrome

A steal phenomenon may be present in the radial artery distal to the anastomosis as blood is drawn toward the low-resistance shunt site rather than progressing toward the hand in a normal manner. This can result in ischemic pain in the hand, although in many cases no symptoms are noted. Determination of the presence of flow reversal is readily accomplished with CCDS making diagnosis of a steal syndrome straightforward. Flow reversal in the distal radial artery may also occur when there is occlusion or high-grade stenosis of the vessel proximal to the anastomosis (Fig. 14). This accounts for the fact that significant arterial compromise proximal to the anastomotic site does not necessarily result in occlusion of the venous limb of the dialysis fistula. A subclavian steal phenomenon with reversed flow in the vertebral artery (see vertebral artery chapter) secondary to a dialysis fistula in the ipsilateral arm has also been described in the literature.

Conclusion

Within certain limitations, CCDS seems to be a useful and promising tool for the diagnostic evaluation of dialysis fistulas. A major advantage of CCDS compared to duplex Doppler sonography is that flow information is available, in real-time, for the entire course of the vessel lumen. This greatly facilitates accurate assessment of even quite tortuous vessels, resulting in an examination which is easier, safer, and more rapidly completed. Even so, the accuracy of the method varies with the nature of the vascular segment being examined and does not fully reach the levels of accuracy attainable with angiography (Table 2). On the positive side, CCDS is a readily available, non-invasive method which can even be used at the patient's

Table 2. Diagnostic values of CCDS for the identification of pathologic alterations of any kind based on 66 examinations with angiographic correlation (from Landwehr et al., 1990)

Veins	Artery	Anastomosis	Vein	Central
Sensitivity (%)	100.0	90.9	97.2	36.4
Specifity (%)	98.1	93.2	93.3	100.0
Accuracy (%)	98.5	92.4	95.5	89.4

bedside. The accuracy of the technique is sufficient to justify its recommendation as a screening method, with angiography reserved for unclear cases or in those instances where surgical or radiologic intervention is planned.

References

Arlart IP, Merk J, Eichner H (1985) DSA mittels Feinnadelpunktion zum Ausschluß vaskulärer Komplikationen bei Hämodialyse-Shunts. Röntgenpraxis 38:200–205

Brescia MJ, Cimino JE, Appel K, et al (1966) Chronic hemodialysis using venipuncture and a surgically created arteriovenous fistula. N Engl J Med 275:1089–1092

Cada E, Karnel F, Mayer G, Längle F, Schurawitzki H, Graf H (1989) Percutaneous transluminal angioplasty of failing arteriovenous dialysis fistulae. Nephrol Dial Transplant 4:57–61

Cimochowski GE, Worley E, Rutherford WE, Sartain J, Blondin J, Harter H (1990) Superiority of the internal jugular over the subclavian access for temporary dialysis. Nephron 54:154–161

Duncan H, Ferguson L, Faris I (1986) Incidence of the radial steal syndrome in patients with Brescia fistula for hemodialysis: Its clinical significance. J Vasc Surg 4:144–147

Erasmi H, Neufang KFR, Schmitz-Rixen Th, de Vleeschauwer Ph, Horsch S (1985) Erfahrungen mit der digitalen Subtraktionsangiographie (DSA) bei Dialyse-Shunt-Komplikationen. Vasa 14:144–148

Glanz S, Gordon DH, Butt KMH, Hong J, Lipkowitz GS (1987) The role of percutaneous angioplasty in the management of chronic hemodialysis fistulas. Ann Surg 206:777–781

Hubsch PJ, Stiglbauer RL, Schwaighofer BW, Kainberger FM, Barton PP (1988) Internal jugular and subclavian vein thrombosis caused by central venous catheters. Evaluation using Doppler blood-flow imaging. J Ultrasound Med 7:629–636

Jameson MD, Wiegmann TB (1990) Principles, uses, and complications of hemodialysis. Med Clin North Am 74:945–960

Kathrein H, König P, Weimann S, Judmaier G, Dittrich P (1989) Nichtinvasive morphologische und funktionelle Beurteilung arteriovenöser Fisteln von Dialysepatienten mit der Duplexsonographie. Ultraschall 10:33–40

Kottle SP, Gonzalez AC, Macon EJ, Fellner SK (1978) Ultrasonographic evaluation of vascular access complications. Radiology 129:751–754

Kotval PS, Shah PM, Berman H (1989) Doppler diagnosis of subclavian steal due to arteriovenous hemodialysis fistula in the ipsilateral arm. J Ultrasound Med 8:697–700

Krpan D, Demarin V, Prot F, Milutinovik S, Molnar V, Milutinovic E (1991). Measurement of blood flow through AV-fistulae by means of Doppler sonography in regularly haemodialysed patients. Int J Artif Organs 14:78–82

Landwehr P, Tschammler A, Schaefer RM, Lackner K (1990) Wertigkeit der farbkodiertem Duplexsonographie des Dialyseshunts. Fortschr Röntgenstr 153:185–191

Langer M, Fiegler W, Claussen C, Köhler D, Banzer D (1984) Arterielle digitale Subtraktionsangiographie zur Darstellung von Hämodialyseshunts. Radiologe 24:576–578

Middleton WD, Erickson S, Melson GL (1989) Perivascular color artifact: pathologic significance and appearance on color Doppler US images. Radiology 171(3):647–652

Middleton WD, Picus DD, Marx MV, Melson GL (1989) Color Doppler sonography of hemodialysis vascular access: Comparison with angiography. AJR 152:633–639

Neufang KFR, Erasmi-Körber H, Wimmer G (1983) Verfahren der Shuntdarstellung bei Dialysepatienten unter besonderer Berücksichtigung der digitalen Subtraktionsangiographie (DSA). Röntgenblätter 36:145–151

Oates CP, Williams ED, McHugh MI (1990) The use of a duplex ultrasound scanner to measure volume flow in arterio-venous fistulae in patients undergoing haemodialysis: an analysis of measurement uncertainties. Ultrasound Med Biol 16:571–579

Picus D, van Breda A, Katzen BT, Steinberg DL (1987) Use of digital subtraction angiography for evaluation of vascular access for hemodialysis. Cardiovasc Intervent Radiol 10:210–214

Pourchez T, Moriniere P, Fournier A, Pietri J (1989) Use of Permcath (Quinton) catheter in Uraemic patients in whom the creation of conventional vascular access for haemodialysis is difficult. Nephron 53:297–302

Quinton W, Dillard D, Scribner BH (1960) Cannulation of blood vessels for prolonged hemodialysis. Trans Am Soc Artif Intern Organ 6:104

Rodriguez-Perez JC, Maynar M, Rams A, et al (1990) Percutaneous transluminal angioplasty as best treatment in stenosis of vascular access for hemodialysis. Nephron 51:192–196

Scheible W, Skram Chr, Leopold GR (1980) High resolution real-time sonography of hemodialysis vascular access complications. AJR 134:1173–1176

Schumcher KA, Wallner B, Weidenmaier W, Friedrich JM (1989) Shuntferne venöse Okklusionen als Störungsfaktoren bei der Hämodialyse. Fortschr Röntgenstr 150:198–201

Schwab SJ, Raymond JR, Saeed M, Newman GE, Dennis PA, Bollinger RR (1989) Prevention of hemodialysis fistula thrombosis. Early detection of venous stenosis. Kidney Int 36:707–711

Tordoir JH, Hoeneveld H, Eikelboom BC, Kitslaar PJ (1990) The correlation between clinical and duplex ultrasound parameters and the development of complications in arterio-venous fistulae for hemodialysis. Eur J Vasc Surg 4:179–184

Tordoir JH, deBruin HG, Hoeneveld H, Eikelboom BC, Kitslaar PJ (1989) Duplex ultrasound scanning in the assessment of arteriovenous fistulas created for hemodialysis access: comparison with digital subtraction angiography. J Vasc Surg 10:122–128

Vanholder R, Hoenich N, Ringoir S (1987) Morbidity and mortality of central venous catheter hemodialysis: a view of 10 years experience. Nephron 47:274–279

Vorwerk D, Günther RW, Bohndorf K, Asgarzadeh A, Borchers K (1988) Farbkodierte Duplexsonographie (Angiodynographie) in der Beurteilung arteriovenöser Shunts. Fortschr Röntgenstr 148:265–268

Windus DW, Audrain J, Vanderson R, Jendrisak MD, Picus D, Delmez JA (1990) Optimization of high-efficiency hemodialysis by detection and correction of fistula dysfunction. Kidney Int 38:337–341

Subject Index

MIX
Papier aus verantwortungsvollen Quellen
Paper from responsible sources
FSC® C105338

If you have any concerns about our products,
you can contact us on
ProductSafety@springernature.com

In case Publisher is established outside the EU,
the EU authorized representative is:
Springer Nature Customer Service Center GmbH
Europaplatz 3, 69115 Heidelberg, Germany

Printed by Libri Plureos GmbH
in Hamburg, Germany